REALITY
FITNESS

REALITY FITNESS

inspiration for your
health and well-being

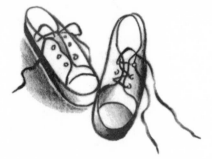

NICKI ANDERSON

NEW WORLD LIBRARY
NOVATO, CALIFORNIA

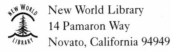

New World Library
14 Pamaron Way
Novato, California 94949

Copyright © 2000 by Nicki Anderson

Cover design and illustration: Kathy Warinner
Text design: Mary Ann Casler

Library of Congress Cataloging-in-Publication Data
    Anderson, Nicki.
    Reality fitness : inspiration for your health and well-being / Nicki
    Anderson.
        p. cm.
    ISBN 1-57731-101-9 (pbk.)
    1. Physical fitness for women. 2. Exercise for women. 3. Women —
    Health and hygiene. I. Title.
RA781.A595 2000
613.7'045—dc21
                                                            99-050089

First printing, March 2000
ISBN 1-57731-101-9
Printed in Canada on acid-free, recycled paper
Distributed to the trade by Publishers Group West

10 9 8 7 6 5 4 3 2 1

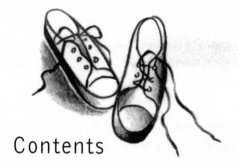

Contents

Acknowledgments

It is never a single hand that completes a book. It is many hands pushing toward creating just the right words that will empower each reader. This book was brought to fruition by my agent, Joe Durepos, and my editor, Jason Gardner, who saw my vision and made it a reality. Thank you also to Mimi Kusch, for her excellent editing.

I want to thank each of my clients current and past, who have taught me so much and stirred me to put words to paper. Your dedication is inspiring.

I want to thank my sister Earline for her words of encouragement and always believing in me, and my children, Wil, Alex, Mitch, and Allison, who complete the circle in my life. Their love is my prized possession. None of this would have ever been possible without the grace of God, for which I feel truly blessed. And, finally, to my husband, Bill: Your unconditional love and support for me has been the driving force behind creating something to be proud of. Thank you for always believing in me (even when you're skeptical). You ground me but never let me fall.

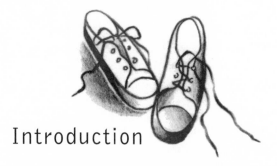

Introduction

LETTING GO!

Junk food is to the body what fad diets are to the mind

I'm fat. Those two short words have dominated my thoughts since I was seventeen. And I'm not alone: Those same words occupy the thoughts of millions of women throughout America. All three girls in my family called themselves fat at some point while growing up. It seemed that no matter what we did, no matter how we starved ourselves, we still came up "fat." Fat as an idea is tenacious. It knows no boundaries. And it's an idea we've created ourselves.

So, what is fat, anyway? Does fat mean cellulite? Does

it mean weighing a few more pounds than we did last year? Does it refer to premenstrual bloating or any loose skin on our thighs? My definition of fat is this: one little word so powerful that, when paired with its partner in crime, the word *diet,* it can completely control our lives. This definition may sound extreme, but then what do you call an 800-calorie-a-day diet? Even the word *fat* stirs up in us such a storm of negative feelings that we lose sight of how tight a grip it has on us. We lose sight of how it leaves us feeling constantly inadequate: We only feel okay about ourselves when the numbers on our scales are "acceptable." So how do we relinquish the hold that our obsessions with fat have on us?

MY STORY

Before becoming a teenager, I never gave my body a second thought. I never worried about whether I was thin or fat. I felt my body was normal — and it was. I was lucky. In the early 1970s, television commercials and magazine ads weren't yet filled with anorexic role models. My thoughts were on growing up, boys, and wanting to fit in. But as I got older, being thin increasingly became a prerequisite to fitting in, and I simply wasn't thin enough. As a result, I slowly lost confidence in how I looked. I began to hide out to eat and felt guilty when someone found me. Eating large family meals was part of my heritage; even that seemed forbidden. To make matters worse, the day I got my driver's license, any exercise I had been getting, like riding my bike, quickly came to a halt. Not only did I stop exercising, but I also discovered the wonderful world of fast food. Now I could simply drive up to a window, order, and get a burger and fries in minutes! A year after I had gotten my license, I was forty-eight pounds heavier. Climbing stairs became hard work, and eating became my favorite pastime. I had become horribly deconditioned at a very young age, and I was miserable. I found myself in a vicious circle. With the extra weight came depression and loneliness. And food proved to be a reliable, comfortable friend. Although I don't, and never will, believe that size dictates health, I watched my self-esteem dwindle along with my physical stamina.

Then I heard about dieting. My first diet at sixteen was moderately successful, according to the almighty scale. I did lose a little weight, but it wasn't enough. Every time I looked in the mirror or stepped on the scale, I was disappointed. I wasn't five foot seven and 105 pounds. I wasn't "ideal." I was seduced by commercials promising that I could be thin and happy if I would just buy into their quick and easy weight-loss plan. Every diet promised sure results. But the diets were never quick and never easy, and nothing is a sure thing. I kept trying these diets, but I never became thin, or my personal definition of thin. The more I dieted, the more a voice in my head whispered, "You're still fat." At first this voice was faint, but it grew as I continued to diet until it became a constant scream.

At that time, I had no clue as to why I was so miserable. I had not yet recognized the need for a positive connection between mind and body. In fact, my mind and body were operating as completely separate entities. The only part of my body I could ever satisfy was my mouth. And that perceived satisfaction resulted in chronic overeating. In retrospect, I believe it was my way of punishing myself for feeling inadequate, so I did it time and again.

Then one day after a holiday meal I began to think about how I felt. Spending two days in recovery from overeating just couldn't be a good thing. I opened myself up and identified how out of sync I felt when I overate. Coming from an inactive, fast-food-imbibing family, I had never learned the importance of fueling your body correctly. I had never learned how partnering quality nutrition with exercise is a necessary component of life at any age. Since I was never particularly athletic, I had little motivation to explore physical activity. But I was beginning to understand that exercise might be a necessary addition to my gradual lifestyle changes. I didn't have a clue where to begin, so I read — voraciously — everything I could find about health. I began to understand that thin is not necessarily fit, that large is not necessarily unfit, and that our bodies are designed to move, move, move. It was an exciting discovery.

THE DESTRUCTION OF DIETS

Each lifestyle change was like a piece of a puzzle. And it took years for all the pieces to fall into place. One of my first attempts at fitting the pieces together was evaluating my nutritional intake. I asked my mother if she would be willing to attend Weight Watchers™ with me, the only safe program available at the time. Unlike other dieting programs, Weight Watchers™ wasn't gimmicky; rather, it provided a strict education on how to eat a well-rounded, balanced diet. As a teen, this information had a great impact on me. Had the program been too restrictive or unbalanced, I never could be where I am today.

With time, I began to understand the connection between eating well-balanced meals and how I felt. What a revelation! At my first weekly meeting, I listened to others' tales about their lack of self-control, which struck a vague chord with me. I had never thought of myself as out of control, but I also knew that I didn't exactly feel *in* control either. I didn't feel in control of my destiny. I wanted to chart a course for a long and happy life. So I began to look at health as simply feeling good and as getting through each day without chastising myself for being fat. Health began with moderation, and in cutting yourself some slack. Slowly but surely, I began to discern the correlation between fueling by body well and feeling this balance.

I began to study further food's effects on the body. I discovered so much through my reading that for the first time I began feeling hopeful about living a life without dieting. My downfall at this point was believing that I knew it all and had total control. Once you finish a diet and achieve your desired result, the diet is "off" and life goes on. I wasn't prepared for that. I figured a year was enough to learn it all and make permanent changes. I was *wrong!* The first sign that I was putting aside all I had learned was my need to weigh myself daily. (Lesson #1: Never weigh yourself every day!) Thinness was becoming more of a goal than health. I became a slave to the numbers on my scale. It happened that fast — all I had pulled together was slipping through my hands.

I had seen a number of ads showing happy, successful women who got it all through diet pills. Why not? I decided to try a diet pill that would block the hunger message and help me eat less. Did it work? You bet, but I was so wired from the pills, I was sleeping three hours a night and in the bathroom the rest of the time dealing with their diuretic effects. And I was eating barely enough to sustain a two-year-old. But, hey, I was thin, and that was what mattered, wasn't it? Yet I had lost what I needed *most* to move forward: reality. I had lost my original goal: to gain control of my health for the long term. I set unrealistic expectations of myself and again bought into what thousands of people do every day: ignore their health and focus on size.

Diets are seductive and destructive, and I fell under their spell. I wanted lower numbers on the scale at any cost. But sneaking Dexatrim™ in my early twenties was no different from sneaking food in my early teens. I was punishing myself for something. Was it for being too good? Or not good enough? Societal messages made it very clear that if you eat too much you're a "loser," but if you're thin, you've got it all together. And sadly, until we get out of its thrall, this is the message we're passing on to the next generation of women.

It was not until I began dating my future husband that I realized how ridiculous my obsession with weight was. Bill never once commented on my size. He accepted all that I was. (Lesson #2: Surround yourself with people who value you.) An even bigger wake-up call came when I became pregnant. I felt so good about the precise care I took of my body that I asked myself, "Why should I value and treat my body well only when I'm pregnant? Why should I return to abusing my body once my child is born?" It was a hard reality check that changed my life. I realized that I valued my baby's health more than my own. And I vowed that day to take better care of myself.

WHY I WROTE THIS BOOK

To return to the question I posed above, how do we release ourselves from the grip that the words *fat* and *diet* have on us? How do we get off the emotional and physical roller coaster we've created? How do we begin focusing on health and rid ourselves of our obsession with numbers — numbers that may or may not be right for us?

I wouldn't be giving you the real scoop if I told you it would be easy. It takes time and patience and awareness — curing ourselves of this obsession really is a kind of rehab. But after years and years of yo-yo dieting, I was fortunate enough to figure out a different approach. It became clear that what I was doing — along with a lot of other women — wasn't working. Like you, I was hoping to discover the great secret that would finally make me perfect. This was all fantasy. In reality, I was a full-time mom with four children under the age of six. I needed to figure out what was appropriate for me — my life, needs, and goals. And I needed to pass a positive message on to my children.

In studying fitness and nutrition, and experimenting with healthy options, I began to discover that nutrition and exercise aren't rocket science. Though the experts lead you to believe that you need them for guidance, you don't! I began to realize that health came partially from eating "whole foods" whenever possible. And for daily movement, I could take the kids for a walk in the stroller when I could manage it. I took the pressure off myself by focusing on reasonable exercise and nutrition. For me that meant finding a way to incorporate regular exercise into my life — without flipping out if it didn't happen that day — and having fun while experimenting with healthy recipes.

It became clear to me that as women, we need to shift our paradigm about diet and exercise and our bodies. We are led to believe that fat equals anything that isn't skinny — really, really skinny. We use the word fat to refer to the slightest bulge or cellulite. Don't misunderstand: some people really are fat, meaning dangerously obese and requiring medical attention, but they're a very small percentage of women. The average woman who thinks of herself as fat isn't. She may be out of shape or have more fat than lean tissue but she is far from dangerously obese. If we are able to shift our paradigm so that fat means being dangerously obese, we'll start to use the term less generally.

We also need to change our perceptions about weight. For too many of us, weight equals numbers on a scale that we let define our mood and who we are. We need to shift that paradigm so that weight is simply a number that fluctuates and varies from body type to body type — a number that isn't necessarily synonymous with health. Generally speaking, there are three very different body types: mesomorph (muscular), ecto-morph (long and lean), and endomorph (full figured). Because of these vastly different body types, no matter what you weigh, no matter how much you diet and exer-cise, your body will not respond the same as *anyone* else. In other words, a mesomorph will never resemble an ecto-morph, and expecting an ectomorph to look like an endo-morph is far from realistic. Evaluate your unique body design and understand both its limitations and potentials.

By shifting these two paradigms — fat and weight — we'll be much less likely to judge who we are by a pant size or scale number. By shifting paradigms, we can begin to look realistically at the probability that you are out of shape or inactive rather than morbidly obese. A unrealistic view of yourself robs you of self-esteem and results in feelings of inadequacy. On the other hand a realistic perspective allows you to choose what to do about a manageable problem.

My goal in writing this book is to help you discern the difference between healthy and unhealthy — that is, between realistic and unrealistic. Putting the word *fat* into perspective can move you forward and allow you to choose a lifestyle that feels right for you. Only then can you feel in charge of your life and begin making deci-sions based on health rather than statistics. That's what *Reality Fitness* is all about: learning to be true to your body and yourself. As I guide you through understanding your own mind-body destiny — the result of becoming more fit — the words *fat* and *diet* will become irrelevant. It won't be easy. Women have been obsessed with thinness for a long time. But *Reality Fitness* will help you release the unrealistic expectations of your past and guide you to realistic ones for your future.

A QUICK HISTORY OF WOMEN'S SELF-EXPECTATIONS

My guess is that women have been body conscious at least as long as they've been fashion conscious — and probably much longer. It's perfectly normal to want to be attractive. But many women have suffered terribly in the name of wanting to look good. The corsets women wore in the nineteenth century to make their waists look tiny sometimes broke their ribs or cut off their breathing. In the 1940s, women were stuffed into fitted, slim-lined skirts, tailored blouses, and snug sweaters. With no other fashion options, plus-size women must have felt like snakes yearning to shed their skin. As a very young girl in the 1960s, I remember my mother and her friends trying every new diet that came along as they tried to be thin like Twiggy and look great in mini-skirts. Every neighbor who gained or lost weight was a topic of discussion. One was notorious for tickling her throat after meals, while another neighbor's unhealthily drastic weight loss — the sad result of a nasty divorce — was envied by all her friends.

Those scenarios haven't changed much over the years. At many social gatherings I've attended, the women end up gathered around the hors d'oeuvre table discussing weight gained and lost or how fat they feel. At a recent coffee klatch, one woman arrived with doughnuts, apologizing that she had only brought them because she was running so late. (After all, eating donuts in public is a no-no!) We all sat around waiting to see who would be the first to grab one of those forbidden treats. Of course no one dared. So the hostess ended up waiting until the last guest left, warmed her coffee, grabbed a doughnut, and enjoyed a moment of bliss. That hostess was me. I admit I hadn't wanted anyone to comment on my lack of control.

When did we relinquish control of our bodies and let societal pressure take over? At what point did we say, They're right and I'm wrong? When did we give up on ourselves? Can women go through a single day without reading, hearing, or seeing an ad for a product or program designed to help you "lose weight the quick and easy way"? Saddest of all is the fact that not one of these ads ever mentions anything about health.

What I eventually discovered was the importance of *overall* health. On my journey back from the diet dungeon, I began to understand the direct correlation between how I felt and eating a balanced diet and exercising moderately. Looking back, missing components from my first attempts at weight loss were exercise, mental and spiritual fulfillment, and a focus on reality. Skinny isn't necessarily an asset; good health is. When I decided to drive less and ride my bike and walk more, I found myself feeling more energetic. When I started appreciating what my body was able to do versus what it couldn't do, I felt better about my abilities. When I was able to take time out to journal and reflect, I felt involved in the moment and grateful for my health.

This is what makes Reality Fitness complete. It isn't just about exercise; it isn't just about nutrition. It's about finding and appreciating just the right things that bring your health and life full circle. It will become clear that anything that leaves you feeling truly good is probably good for you — eating reasonably feels better than overeating, walking for half your lunch hour leaves you feeling better than sitting in your office all day. And it's good for your body, mind, and self-esteem. I know it's what worked for me as I learned to respect my body and all it had to offer.

After this discovery, I decided my mission in life was to educate women and teens about their exercise options. Going back to school to become a Certified Personal Fitness Trainer and Fitness Practitioner has allowed me to do that. After ten years of experience teaching various fitness regimes, plenty of reading and studying, trial and error, I have much to pass on to you, both personally and professionally. Over the years as a health and fitness motivational speaker, I have had the opportunity to present seminars to hundreds of women, all of whom were reaching aimlessly toward an unrealistic goal. It is my hope that with this book, I will help you set realistic fitness goals for yourself and give you the opportunity to meet them.

CHOOSING HEALTH OVER THINNESS

First, recognize your gene pool. It's time to say, "Thanks Mom, thanks Dad," and move on. You cannot reconfigure your genes; you are who you are. I have short, olive-skinned parents. No program on earth is going to make me tall and fair. No matter how hard I try, that's just not part of who I am. Once you begin to accept who you are, you are able to set more realistic goals for yourself. Knowing what is realistic and what you can actually attain through a healthy lifestyle generates motivation. Look at a newsstand full of fashion magazines. The cover models are beautiful; their big incomes depend on it. Unless you're a model, your job doesn't depend on how thin you are or how perfect your hair is. We all like to feel good about how we look, but we continue to misplace our emphasis on the things we can't change. Let's begin now by letting go of who society impels us to be and explore what we really want and what is right for us.

One of my clients summed this point up perfectly when she told me, "When I started thinking yet again about a diet or being thin, the whole idea really turned me off. I'm tired of it and can't do it anymore. So I started thinking about being healthy. That sparked hope for me. I can be as healthy or unhealthy as I want and gauge it all on my own. That's exciting!" For her, turning away from the pitfalls of dieting gave her an opportunity to set realistic goals and to be successful in meeting them. Rather than walking to procure a thin waist, she started walking to have a stronger heart, stronger legs, and a better sense of the beauty surrounding her. If you walk just to reach an unrealistic goal, such as having a thirteen-inch waist, you'll soon give up. If you walk because it makes a positive difference in how you feel, more than likely it will become a lifelong habit.

I can't stress it enough: Health is how we feel about ourselves, not being a perfect size two (and many size twos are in reality dangerously malnourished). And creating a healthy lifestyle *will not only* change our perspective but bring us closer to our goal of becoming fit. We waste so much precious time focusing on our imperfections that we fail to notice what makes each of us so uniquely *us*. How long do you agonize over the fact that you ate a piece of chocolate? How many times have you gone to the doctor's office and been aghast when you weighed five pounds more than you did at home? Do you let that number wreck your day? How many times have you gone out to dinner with friends and then beat yourself up because you cleared your plate? I know I used to.

Imagine all the extra time we would all have if we focused on the boundless capabilities of our bodies and minds rather than on our inadequacy or our measurements. Say we waste a good ten minutes every hour every day mentally chastising ourselves about what we eat, how we look, and so forth. Based on a fifteen-hour day — not counting our dream time — that adds up to almost three hours a day! What if you spent those hours realizing how great you feel about where you are in your life right now? About the opportunity to make some great changes? That is where health and fitness start coming together. By incorporating healthful choices, each choice draws you toward a higher level of fitness, because fitness is really the union of nutrition, movement, mind, and spirit.

Essentially, if we despise our bodies we are despising the gifts that get us through each day. We are taking for granted the house that bears children, feels love, tells stories, and hugs tight. We're condemning the flesh and bones that enable us to walk in a park, move to our favorite songs, and feel the chill of winter on our cheeks. If we are not happy with the house that holds the gift of life, then we are sadly limiting all the joy that is possible during our short stay on this planet. Why not look ahead and rejoice in all that life has to offer? As you learn how to face reality and *learn to love the body you're in*, you will reveal the unlimited joy and peace that can fill your life. So I invite you, with enthusiasm, passion, and determination, to let go of all the limitations you've placed on yourself and embrace who you truly are.

Close your eyes for a moment and focus on all the parts of your body that are uniquely yours: blue eyes, hazel eyes, brown eyes, long hair, short hair, curly hair. These are our true gifts that make each of us so magnificent. Our bodies are amazing creations. You may have unique eyes or thick silky hair — no two people are alike. We are singular, and that is cause for celebration.

Today is the day to let go and begin to understand what makes life truly full. It is our responsibility to create a healthy future for ourselves and the up-and-coming weight-conscious girls who think there is no life without a perfect figure. It's time to get excited about the possibilities and feel good about who we are and not what our bathroom scale says. Only then can we create a healthy, exciting future for ourselves.

Reality Fitness will take you from diet disasters to a new way of life — a way to look at life realistically through a lens of health and happiness rather than one of disappointment and hopelessness. With the guidance of this book, you can begin to experience a success that no diet in the world can provide. Fad diets focus solely on the body. They set you up for failure and erode self-respect. With Reality Fitness, good health results from a strengthened body, a nurtured spirit, and a well-fed mind. These components complete the circle of health and bring success. And with that success comes plain old fitness. Begin by accepting where you are now, and think about where you want to go — physically, mentally, and spiritually. Then let go and discover all you can be.

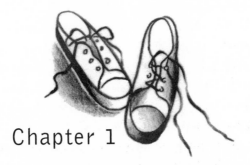

Chapter 1

WHAT IS FITNESS?

Thin and fit are no more related than smart and sensible

Fitness equals thinness — that seems to be the consensus among Americans today. As American women starve themselves to look like the cover of the latest fashion magazine, they believe they're fit. When others see the latest "muscle fitness" magazines displaying "six-pack" abs and people with muscles in places where I don't believe muscles are even supposed to be, they then believe *that* is fit!

Our understanding of the word *fitness* continues to be narrowly defined and mistakenly perceived. Many believe that fitness is only available to those willing to climb Mount

Everest or to run a marathon. Unfortunately, for many of us, the word *fitness* has been linked strictly to physical appearance or athletic prowess — and always a little bit out of reach. If you're very active, you might consider being fit the same as being a professional athlete. If you're moderately active, you may define fit as someone who exercises three times a week. If you're completely sedentary, you probably define fit as being able to get out of bed every morning. What's most important is that we *not* define being fit as the impossible. Fitness is attainable by anyone who desires to be healthy!

FITNESS FOR ALL!

My dictionary defines *fit* as "suitable, strong, appropriate, happy." That encompasses far more than just the physical, yet we consistently view fitness as a state of physical perfection, instead of viewing it as our state of overall well-being. I define *fitness* as simply a kind of mental, spiritual, and physical synergy, as a blend of components that allow your body to work at its optimum. The challenge is figuring out how to bring those components together to achieve wholeness or wellness, that is, fitness. Bringing those components together is what Reality Fitness is all about.

Becoming fit involves more than just pumping iron or walking every day. Fitness begins with exploring which part of your life seems most out of sync and then figuring out what you are willing to do to straighten it out. Because fitness encompasses body, mind, and spirit, we must make exercise part of our lives to bolster our physical fitness. As we improve our physical fitness we are better able to complete daily tasks with less effort, and overall energy improves to enhance the quality of our lives. Physical fitness "opens the flood gates" to a better quality of life. Fitness boosts awareness about all that your body is capable of both physically and mentally.

When I give my seminars, I often ask women how they define fitness. The common response is "skinny" or "athletic." But some of the most fit people I know would never be selected out of a crowd as being fit. Why? Because they don't have the stereotypically buff or thin body we readily recognize as fit. Rather, they are fit by virtue of their strong minds, strong bodies, and strong sense of who they are.

I was reminded how easily we fall into the narrow definition of fitness when I made the decision to run the Chicago marathon. When first considering it, I found myself caught in my old thoughts of "being fit means being athletic" trap. A friend kept encouraging me to do my long-distance runs with a group of area runners. I didn't want to because I felt they'd all be in "really good shape," while I was only a first-time long-distance runner. My friend's persistence paid off, and I finally agreed to run. At the marathon, I was pleasantly surprised to see runners of all sizes, shapes, and ages. They were warm, encouraging, and fun. The truth is that everyone present was in shape, but not just physically; they seemed complete. The mental and spiritual state of the runners there was obvious as they cheered others on and showed concern for those struggling. The marathon was a wonderful experience that I remember whenever I catch myself falling back into equating fitness with physical perfection. Again, fitness not only includes body strength but mental and spiritual strength as well.

So here's one way to keep in mind a new definition of fit: **F** Feeling **I** Incredibly **T** Terrific. It may sound corny, but you know how good you feel when everything feels right and you feel energized and ready to take on the world. If you don't, you soon will!

CHARTING YOUR FITNESS JOURNEY

Begin by examining how you live your life every day. It's important to understand that your level of fitness is your own to decide. If you hate to run, why make yourself go running every day? Do you like leisurely walks in the park? Riding your bike with a friend? Make your activity something that you look forward to. You have to do things that feed all aspects of who you are. An exercise you don't like will affect your mind and spirit negatively. Your choice needs to resonate with all of you, not just your physical self.

Discovering which activities are just right for you is half the battle. Some people never find anything they like because if it's not what professional athletes do, they believe it's not going to be effective. If you've been walking faithfully every day and you feel energized and strong, then that is fit for you. What's important is that you're doing *something*, and that that something fits *you*.

Most clients who come to my studio are interested in losing weight. Then they happen to mention they want to increase their energy level and basically feel better. My response is, "Oh, you want to be fit." They give me a confused look and say, "Oh, no, I just want to be a little stronger and feel better." So then I tell them, "That is what fitness is. Being fit isn't a destination, it's an ongoing process of discovery. The discovery of what brings out the best in you." For those clients, this statement is a real revelation. They've always looked at people who were athletic, thin, or visibly chiseled as fit, never dreaming that a positive state of mind and body are both by-products of becoming fit and actually a possibility in their lives.

The main problem with defining fitness too narrowly is that your exploration into other fitness arenas will be cut short. In other words, if you focus too much on becoming a perfect size six, you might think that an hour and a half of power walking is the only way to reach that goal. In turn you will overlook wonderful options such as taking tennis lessons or walking with your kids, which can lead you just as well to another level of fitness and, as a by-product, possibly a smaller size. The fewer choices you feel are available, the harder it will be to find just the right fitness program.

During the initial stages of planning your fitness program, choose your first step carefully. It's important that you don't overwhelm yourself with too many things at once. If you're trying to start an exercise program, keep it simple. Gradually *(gradually* being the key word here) introduce something new until you feel you've mastered it, then proceed to the next level either with the same activity or by moving on to another fitness challenge. For example, if you have been completely sedentary, I would not encourage you to walk for an hour every day. Start with ten minute walks, three times a week. Once you have mastered that, either add on another day or five minutes to your current days. The idea is to set goals that are attainable. People often raise the bar too high, can't make it over, and quit in frustration.

If you decide (after years of being sedentary) to become a long-distance runner, go for it! Just understand it can't be done overnight. Realize that becoming a distance runner demands time, dedication, and hard work. Evaluate how realistic your goal and timeline is. Don't set yourself up for failure. If some day you would like to walk or run a five-kilometer race (3.2 miles), your approach to nutrition and exercise will be different from the woman who wants to train for a fifty-mile bikeathon. This doesn't mean that you are any less fit than she is. In the end, you're both working on creating a healthier self. Exercise involves reaching an acceptable physical state that is appropriate and attainable for you. Focus on the outcome of your program so you can better visualize your fitness success. That successful outcome is the message you need to feed your mind every day.

Envision what *you* believe fit to be. How does it feel? Strong, contented, energized? If you're currently inactive, for you, fitness might begin with walking around the block for fifteen minutes. If you've already been walking, you might want to expand your program to include walking a mile in less than fifteen minutes. The point is to do something more than you're doing now to keep your body, spirit, and mind strong. You may not be able to walk out your door tomorrow and start a power walking session, but that doesn't matter. What matters is that you're doing *something*, today.

Fitness can begin at any age. Don't let the fact that you've just turned fifty stop you from becoming more active or from jumping into something new such as rock climbing, water aerobics, or getting a couple of friends together for a daily power walk (always remembering to check with your physician if you've been inactive). As our bodies go through the natural aging process you may never attain that "flat tummy." (What makes it so necessary anyway?) Or maybe that bottom hangs a little lower than it used to. That doesn't exempt you from being fit. Your body changes; it's part of the process. Accept it, appreciate all you can do, and delight in the possibilities! You can take some of the pressure off yourself by not trying to reach some goal that has nothing to do with being healthy and strong: a flat tummy doesn't guarantee a strong cardiovascular system, which is much more important. Embrace the wonderful freedom that will allow you to mature with grace, beauty, and strength.

Without question, as we age our fitness options may fluctuate. Making time for fitness becomes far more challenging in our thirties and forties as we're building our futures, raising our kids, advancing our careers, and so forth. Many of us put our own needs aside to help everyone else out. Be careful about always focusing on everyone else's needs. Sure, as parents sometimes we need to give up some "me" time, but it's important not to give it up completely. Keeping an appointment time for your fitness regime doesn't have to take hours out of a day. Ten minutes here, fifteen minutes there can feed the psyche and change your life. Remember that if you want to be a giving wife, manager, mother, friend, leader, partner, and so forth, you can't give if your pockets are empty.

Speaking for myself, when I'm busy at work and my kids' demands for help with their homework is at a peak, I wonder when I'll ever get a minute to take a stress-relief walk or to read a chapter in an inspiring book. I have had to learn how to balance the different parts of my life so that I don't become so overwhelmed that I lose all I've worked so hard to achieve. If I spread myself too thin, all areas of my life suffer, and in the end the one who suffers the most is me. Part of my mental fitness program is learning what I can reasonably take on and what I must turn down. For women in particular, saying "no" can be very hard. Many of us have been trained to put others' needs in front of our own. Today I welcome the chance to say "no" to what I don't wish to do and "yes" to what I desire — without any more explanation than a simple "yes" or "no." Anything less than that would be selling myself short. It's important to focus your sights on what is reasonable. Practice telling your boss that you can't stay late to help out, then go home and take that lovely evening walk.

Being fit lies along a spectrum from walking up and down stairs to do the laundry to training for a triathlon. Your program will depend on what your needs are and what your lifestyle can accommodate, so listen closely to yourself. As I've stated before, *being* fit isn't a prerequisite to *getting* fit. I've had clients tell me, "Being fit is for athletes, not for a mom at home with three kids." That couldn't be further from the truth. More than ever a mother with children needs some time for release and a quiet mind. Feeding your mind and body with activities that leave you feeling in sync is the key. If you run every day yet don't get adequate sleep, if you only eat fast food and never feed your mind anything new, then you are not really fit. On the other hand, if you get a good night's sleep, generally eat healthful foods, and feed your mind with good books, then you're more fit that the marathon runner who lives on junk food.

Fitness is not made up of the single component of exercise. So strengthening your body through exercise is just as important as taking the time to do something that grounds you. Maybe going to museums on the weekend or getting together with a girlfriend for lunch. These "activities," though not exercise, are exercises in self-preservation and building health. If all you do is physical exercise and you never do things to calm the spirit and fuel the mind you'll feel incomplete. The marriage of exercise to other pleasurable activities is what brings true fitness.

So, let's shift our thoughts from leaping tall buildings in a single bound to walking every day. Let's switch from going after sculpted abs to having strong abs to prevent low back injuries. And let's stop spending money on fad diets in an attempt to reach a "perfect" weight. Once we're able to contemplate that shift, we'll realize that fitness really just entails being happy and productive rather than lethargic and frustrated.

When I walk into a room to give a seminar, I often hear many sighs of relief. Why? Because I don't fit the mold of the traditional "fitness" person. Many people tell me they equate fitness with a blonde bombshell or with Arnold Schwarzenegger. I am brunette and average in build, and I am happy with that. I know that I move my body daily with exercise, take time to meditate, and read at least one thing a day that educates or motivates me toward good health. So though I may not fit the bill of the "fitness guru," I feel fit, intellectually, physically, and spiritually. That's what matters to me.

WHERE DOES FITNESS START?

So you're ready to chart your fitness journey. The more clarity you have about your journey, the more likely that you will be able to embark and proceed successfully. Begin by asking yourself, "Why do I want to be fit?" It's vital that you are able to answer that question so you are better able to understand your goals. Remember, there's no right or wrong answer; asking yourself this question simply provides an opportunity for you to think about the course of your path toward enriching your life. The answer to the question might be that you want to improve your energy level or prevent heart disease. Maybe you feel the need for some mental or spiritual inspiration. Or you may just be tired of feeling "draggy" all the time and would like to commit to being more *proactive* with your health, proactive being the key word here. You cannot attain any level of fitness unless you take an active role in sorting out what you need and don't need to make your journey a success.

As you begin your journey, here are some important tips to bear in mind. Let's say that you've decided to walk every day. Or maybe you're already walking every day but stressing out about how to fit walking into your daily routine. Let me say that becoming fit when you're stressed out is rather incongruent. How can you develop a fit lifestyle when you're stressed and frustrated? Perhaps this analogy will help. When you think of fitness, think of weeding a garden. What do you do? You throw away the weeds that are of no use, while nurturing the things that will grow and bloom and add beauty to your garden. When seeking proper fitness through balance you can adopt the same strategy. Keep what moves you forward mentally, physically, and spiritually and cast aside the things that keep you stagnant or pull you down. For example, do you have friends or family who make fun of your fitness efforts? Or maybe they encourage you to "have fun" instead of going for a walk or reading a good book. I have often found that when you're on the road to success, there are those, even those who are very close to you, who may try to sabotage your efforts. One way of casting aside those things that pull you down is to associate less with those who do not respect your good intentions so that you'll be better equipped to move ahead, ever so slowly, as you grow more comfortable with the idea of creating a healthier you by becoming fit.

After you've asked yourself the question, "Why do I want to be fit," the next step is to assess your thoughts and actions throughout the day and evaluate how you feel at day's end. When I went through this process, I was amazed at how my overloaded life still missed some important things. I'd get up at 6:00 A.M. to get the kids off to school, then I'd go to work, come home, cook supper, help the kids with their homework, do some laundry, then read bedtime stories to the kids. I began to explore the missing elements in my daily routine. For example, I found that reading for fifteen minutes before bed every night helped soothe my mind and fill me with positive images to fall asleep with. I also discovered that I can wake up a half hour earlier to take a walk, while cherishing the silence. In other words, it doesn't take much. Fifteen minutes well spent can be life-altering food for the body and soul. I also discovered the very important benefits of journaling. I believe it's what makes or breaks a successful program.

JOURNAL YOUR WAY TO FITNESS

As I've mentioned before, fitness is forever. With my clients as well as myself, success seems to follow those that commit to journaling. Journaling is the best way to keep your thumb on the pulse of your day-to-day challenges and successes. Initially the idea of writing things down is yet another thing to add to an already tight schedule. I have found, however, that those who journal are actually able to create more clarity and organization in their lives. So I encourage you to get comfortable with the idea of journaling first. If you're a detail person, write as much as you need. If you want to be short and sweet, that's fine also. First, find a journal with special meaning. Carefully select the color or the picture on the cover and the size of the journal. Make it right for you. Then begin to document your evolution toward healthy living. It's wonderful to look back and see where you started and how far you've come. You are better able to center yourself when you can see your progress and review the challenging times and how you overcame them.

When you've selected just the right journal, find a quiet spot for writing. Begin with closing your eyes and seeing yourself as fit. What do you see yourself doing? Are you hiking up a beautiful mountain? Are you playing hopscotch with your children? Are you going for a long walk with a good friend? Maybe you're meditating while concentrating on proper breathing? What did you see? Write it down, and list the details. Where were you? Were you alone? What do you see when you're done creating your vision of fitness? Are you refreshed? Do you look content? Happy? Sweaty? Was it good to see yourself like that? Maybe you had a hard time deciding what you might do to be fit. That too is a step forward as you familiarize yourself with your personal definition of fitness. It's best to think about it for a while, to let what you've read sink in and your thoughts continue a bit before you dive in. For some, it's quite an eye opener when they discover that being fit doesn't involve hours of brutal exercise with pounding music in the background, but rather a beautiful journey toward the recognition of all that is possible.

INCH BY INCH

Be patient with yourself as you sort out exactly what's missing in your life and find new ways to provide yourself with those things. Your goal is to create personal peace and balance. There will be occasions when your body and mind don't seem to jibe, but that doesn't mean you're doing something wrong. You may just be having an off day. You're sick, or the kids are sick, or you're overwhelmed as you prepare for some holiday festivity. And we mustn't forget PMS, which can take us from feeling great to feeling like the world has come to an end and it's all our fault!

Life can be so hectic and can involve so many pressures that we often fail to realize how much of our energy, both physical and mental, is drained. Any major event, positive or negative, can make a huge impact on our daily lives, sometimes for a day, sometimes for a month, sometimes for a year, and sometimes forever. One reason it is so important to maintain your fitness level is so that you have more peace and strength with which to meet these major events. When you feel you've lost control, you can always go for a walk, meditate quietly for even a few minutes, or do some deep breathing in an effort to get yourself back in sync. Some women with whom I've worked who suffer from PMS notice a marked difference when they meditate, stretch, and do aerobic activity daily. Those elements bring about complete fitness, which is a natural remedy in its simplest form.

Life isn't always meant to be easy, but it is meant to be full. It's up to you to concentrate on the fullness of life so that you'll be better equipped to handle any obstacles that may come your way. Even if you can only fit in meditation during your child's nap time or during a coffee break, the point is to fit it in. That couple of minutes you take may be the difference between flying off the handle or sitting back and understanding that whatever has upset you may not be that big a deal.

We all know that life can't be great all the time, so don't make yourself crazy trying to make it so. After all, we're talking about *Reality* Fitness! The best you can do each day is to keep mind, body, and spirit acquainted with one another. The more you achieve this kind of unity, the greater the likelihood you have of attaining long-term wellness and fitness.

I often remind my clients, "Do what you can to be as fit as you can today, because it will all change within the year." Our ever-changing lives and the curve balls that are thrown our way confirm that change is constant. Still, with all that changes in our lives, every New Year (as we're all trying to get a life back after the holidays) we dive into an Ironman training program in an attempt to retrieve our twenty-year-old bodies, believing that's what it will take to get our lives back in balance. We then add insult to injury when after six weeks we're disappointed that we're not sporting that great body and feeling terrific. Often, because that unrealistic goal wasn't achieved, we forgo any other efforts to improve the quality of our lives.

This is where we get into trouble by narrowly defining fitness. Everyone thinks that going to the gym will make everything better. I know — and now you know — it won't. The problem lies in placing all of our efforts on the outside and nothing on the inside. I don't know about you, but after the holidays, I need some down time. I need time to regroup and be kind to myself and nurture the part of me that really needs attention, my spirit and mind. Only then am I able to start understanding what my body needs and then add it in to my fitness regime. Ask yourself what it is that you need to get yourself centered? What part of yourself have you lost touch with?

Starting this excursion toward being fit may be easy for some. For those of you who have been inactive, give yourself adequate time to figure it out. Rome wasn't built in a day and your habits didn't evolve over the last month. Allow this metamorphosis to take time. You may need to finish reading this book to get a full understanding of all that you've kept yourself from doing thus far. Make comfortable choices about your activity level. As I mentioned earlier, there is no right or wrong, and no one is judging what you do.

Your body, mind, and spirit are the sole beneficiaries of all that you do. So make positive choices understanding that there will be some bumps in the road—what road doesn't have bumps? What makes Reality Fitness so refreshing is that it's about real life and setting reasonable goals for yourself and being comfortable with those choices. It's a journey that will enhance your life, your future — all because you're able to provide yourself with building blocks of long-term health. Look to the future with great anticipation as you become strong, healthy, and fit!

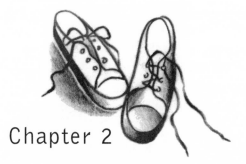

Chapter 2

THE BALANCING ACT

Only through balance is one able
to blend body, mind, and spirit,
bringing forth fitness in its truest form

Can you recall the times when you have felt completely at peace? How about when you've felt comfortable in your body and content with your life? If you're like most people, those moments rarely occur as you rush to keep pace with an overly busy life that now feels completely normal. For me, an ongoing challenge is to find a moment to sit and appreciate pure simplicity and serenity.

Unfortunately the times that stand out in my mind are those chaotic days when I'm pulling my hair out and longing for the day to end. I believe that's the reality for most of us.

How did the meaningful times get lost in the busy, difficult times? What has happened that we have so little time for anyone or anything — including ourselves? In this age of technology, we often seem oblivious to all that's been left behind, including a simpler, more valued life.

Sometimes it feels like all work and no play, even for our children. If we're not running to catch the train for work, we're driving the kids to some activity or we're attending meetings and making schedules. We're checking voice mail, e-mail, and plain old mail. Something's got to give, lest we detonate from sheer overload. It is time to evaluate where we are in our lives, to prioritize and to stabilize. We all know we want to make some changes, but just knowing that we need to change does not mean that we are able to get past the "should do" list. We've got millions of excuses!

But like anything else in life, if you want something badly enough, you have to be willing to make sacrifices. If you have a deep desire to change and enhance your life, you can do it. You must simply envision the outcome and then approach your decision to make changes head on. Some people may need to hit bottom before they're able to accept that changes need to be made. Others may decide to change when they simply wake up one morning feeling like life is passing them by and ask, "Where did the time go?"

Many of us have reached the point of wishing we had listened more to our loved ones, exercised more, read more, and so forth. If you believe that your life is moving too quickly and that you're losing control, then it's time to stop, reevaluate, and decide what you can do *now* to bring some peace and balance to your life. It's never too late to make positive changes. Initially, thoughts of change can be very overwhelming. To keep things in perspective, draw up a plan for change one step at a time — breaking change into smaller, more manageable pieces.

You can begin by determining what aspects of your life you're able to change now and what can be dealt with down the road. If you are in a state of constant stress you need to pinpoint its cause. Is it involving yourself in too much at work? Is it volunteering for too many things? Are you always tired because you eat on the run and are never able to get any exercise? Sit back and determine what things must go in order to bring some sanity to your life. Sometimes we get so caught up in all we're doing we don't even realize what it's doing to us. Too much stress, too little exercise, too many deadlines, and too little sleep add up to poor health and poor fitness. As discussed in the previous chapter, to achieve balance, you need to focus on the mind (feeding your mind positive messages daily), care for your body (engaging in physical activity), and nurture the spirit (giving of your time or exploring talents). Only then can you pull it all together and work toward inner and outer balance — fitness.

I don't want to give the impression that a state of balance is a constant; it's not. As I've said, it can be a constant challenge to keep some balance in our lives. The good news is that the longer you work at the things that keep you in balance — working out, writing poetry, journaling — the easier it becomes. Let's begin by taking a look at how you can use your mind, body, and spirit focus so that you're better equipped to create a positive, healthy lifestyle for yourself.

THE MIND: WHAT MESSAGES DO YOU FEED YOURSELF?

For those of us who have experienced the sabotage of our true essence through dieting disasters, it's time we understood how that whole process evolved. I'm not trying to get scientific here. I'm strictly sharing with you how my years of working with hundreds of women and my own experiences have brought me to the following conclusions. Let's return briefly to my teen years, back before I had begun to think of myself as "fat." As a young teen, I never viewed myself as overweight. But when I was a junior in high school, some students there called me "Bertha" in the hallways as I walked by, which was what the guys called the girls they deemed to be overweight. They obviously had their own ideas of what being overweight meant, which I was not privy to. The more they called me this name, the more I began to internalize the name and believe it. I began comparing myself to others. And the more I compared myself to the "skinny" girls, the more I talked myself into the fact that I must really be fat after all. Soon, instead of appreciating who I was becoming as a young woman and respecting my strengths, I started to focus on my protruding belly and my size-fourteen pants. Coupled with the fact that my home life was in crisis, I was talking myself into becoming a failure. Let me repeat that: *I* was talking myself into becoming a failure.

As I fed myself more negative messages, I fed my body negative fuel. In other words, the more depressed I became, the more I ate. It was a vicious cycle, just as it is for millions of women. In retrospect, overeating was my way of punishing myself for having an imperfect body. All I would need to do, and again, I'm certainly not alone in this, is to see a svelte, beautiful woman on the cover of a magazine, and boom! I would feel like a failure and continue feeding myself negative messages.

As a depressed teen, I really did want to improve my life. But at that time, losing weight was my ticket to a perfect life! Like everyone, I was conditioned to believe that. And although I may have been a little overweight due to my inactivity, I allowed the extra weight to be responsible for everything I felt I wasn't. I had gone from feeling quite confident about myself to feeling completely inadequate. As time went on, I allowed those who knew me least to have the most power over my feelings and how I viewed myself — like the diet industry. I had convinced myself I was a loser, unable to make my own decisions and that I needed help, regardless of where that help came from. This is how the thinking goes for so many of us. If you're "fat" you're a failure, and if you're a failure you have no control. If you have no control, you need help, and what do you know? And *voilà,* there's the diet industry ready to escort you into the land of svelte, problem-free living. I fell for it, hook, line, and sinker. All the negative comments people made, all the negative things I believed about myself, became an overload of garbage crowding my mind. What happens when you have a surplus of mental garbage? You've got to find a way to dump it, and I was not doing that.

How many times do you have negative thoughts about your dress size? How many times have you gone to the pool, looked at all the skinny women there, and then left your shirt on for the day? This constant barrage of negative messages creates a huge obstacle to moving forward. Wouldn't it feel great if the next time you saw a TV commercial showing a woman working out with six-pack abs and perky breasts you said to yourself, "Imagine the time she has to spend to get her stomach like that? She's probably never had kids!" The more you are able to keep positive messages in mind, the better able you are to separate what is reality and what is not. Right now your self-perspective is unrealistic. You see yourself as a failure with no way out. You rarely, if ever, like what you see in the mirror.

I can't tell you how many women come to my studio and first thing announce, "I've been bad!" These women don't realize that the more they say such things, the more these messages become ingrained in their minds. I tell them that not getting around to exercising may result in their having less energy or in feeling grumpy, but it does not make them bad. So many of us believe we are inadequate because we've broken some cardinal diet or exercise rule. The end result is that many women end up buried so deeply in negative messages about themselves that they can't see a way out — until now.

When you begin to feed yourself positive messages, you will be able to view yourself in a very different light. If you're buying yourself a size-twelve skirt, and you used to wear a size eight, instead of snarling at yourself in the dressing-room mirror, why not tell yourself how great you look in that color? If you're about to go to your high school reunion and feel horrified that you don't weigh what you did in high school, why not instead focus on how healthy, happy, and accomplished you feel? If you're telling yourself that you should look just like Demi Moore when you just had a baby two weeks earlier, why not instead commend yourself for taking such good care of yourself and your baby in the midst of chaos? The more you rid yourself of negative talk and replace it with positive reinforcing messages, the more you'll be able to make healthy decisions about what's best for you.

Why not start each day feeding yourself confident messages that will bring you up rather than down? When you hear yourself starting to make some condescending inner comment, stop and replace it with something positive. Then, at the end of each day, remind yourself of how many times you were able to avoid negative messages by replacing them with positive ones. Creating positive messages will be challenging at first, since we're not used to doing it. We've spent so much time learning to condemn all that we aren't, that it will be tough at first learning to appreciate all that we are. It will also be a wonderful revelation. Our minds are fertile places and take in much more than we realize. Why not start allowing only those thoughts that will encourage and support you and delete the rest. By doing that you are acting as your personal quality-control manager, making sure you're giving yourself the best. After all, don't you deserve it? The answer is yes!

LOVE THE BODY YOU'RE IN

As long as women strive for figures that are simply unrealistic for them because of their body type, they will fail. As long as they strive to be four dress sizes smaller than they are, they will fail. As long as they strive to look like some videotape cover model, they will fail, over and over again. So many of us have become our own worst enemies.

On an average day, I see about eight clients, each of them dissatisfied with their bodies and seeking a shape that because of genetics they will never attain. These women are unable to see the potential of the bodies they were given. We have been convinced that our bodies should resemble a Barbie doll. What some of us do to our bodies in an attempt to fit in is downright scary. We starve, binge, purge, "suck-n-tuck" — whatever it takes — without worrying about how all these methods will affect us down the road. We are harming perfectly sound bodies to reach something that will never be realistic for us. We need to take into consideration our diversity in genetic makeup, which dictates, among other things, our size, shape, and bone structure. This genetic makeup is the code that creates a one-of-a-kind "us."

When I finally discovered that there was more to me than just my body, it was truly an epiphany. By that I mean I recognized that my unique body type wasn't bad or good, fat or skinny — it was just my body. And accepting my body meant accepting me. I learned that my body is simply an outer reflection of all that I do to care for myself — the accumulation of positive thoughts, nutritious food, and plenty of daily activity. Most important, I began to understand that my body is a home for my mind and spirit, and the better care I give my body, the more I thrive.

So stop listening to the voices telling you how you should look and begin concentrating on what makes your body strong, graceful, and healthy. It's as simple as this: If you are doing all that you can to be healthy, respecting your body by giving it what it needs, that is, healthful fuel and daily exercise, you're doing all you can to be healthy. Just because your body doesn't respond to your efforts by miraculously shrinking down to a size two doesn't mean you've failed. It simply means that your body is where it needs to be for you.

We tell our kids that they don't have to be like everyone else, yet that's precisely what we're trying to do when we try to live by the guidelines set by the diet and fashion industries. But if you abuse, neglect, and obsess about your body, it will never be good enough or small enough to make you feel that you fit in. At my studio, our tag line is, "Love the Body You're In™," and love it you must.

As we enter this new millennium, let's delight in all our bodies are capable of rather than punishing them for what we perceive they are not. Let's appreciate the fact that our bodies are what carry us through each day and that the more we respect them, the more we will receive from life. Begin today to discover what makes you distinctly beautiful and special and I'm sure it's more than one thing! Learn to appreciate the miracle of your body and then treat it well so that in turn it can provide you with years of increased energy and mobility so you are able to take those trips you've wanted to take, play with your kids more, and get involved with physical activities you never thought were possible

NURTURING OUR SPIRITS

As I contemplated writing this section, I was somewhat hesitant. After all, nurturing of spirit has been a very hot topic and, for some, overdone. It also can be a very personal issue. But in the end, I'm glad that we're finally addressing and becoming more attentive to our spirits. And although spirituality is not my area of expertise, I do strongly believe that without mentioning the importance of sustaining spirit, I wouldn't be sharing what I believe to be a vital cog in the wheel of fitness.

When I think of the word *spirit*, the first image I have is that of children and their free spirits. Children are able to use their imaginations, love freely, forgive and forget. I believe we all start out with a spirit that desires to be nurtured. When we are children, that spirit is alive and well, but as we grow older, it often starts to fade. As we enter the teen years, our spirit begins a hibernation process. We lose much of our innocence, we trust less, we love less, and we conform more to society's demands. Sadly, as adults with increasingly busy lives, many of us continue to lose track of our true selves and become vulnerable to outside messages. Being full of spirit means listening to your heart's desires without the pressures of the environment around you. I firmly believe that the body-obsession craze has contributed to many a broken or buried spirit among adult women. So how do we rediscover or glue back together the pieces of the spirit?

Like everything we've discussed so far, it takes sitting down and evaluating where you are, what is missing, and what *you* need to begin putting the fitness puzzle together. As women we are often taught to nurture others but rarely how to nurture ourselves. We will do anything for friends and family, but when it comes to our own needs we just can't find the time. Some of my clients tell me they feel that exercising is selfish because it takes away too much time from the family. I remind them that if you give, give, give to everyone all the time, what's left for you? And if you're left with nothing, you have nothing good to pass on. I also remind them as parents they need to be good role models, and if you love your body enough to take good care of it, you're setting a great example for your children.

In fact, some of the most giving people I know are those who are most content with themselves. When I have moments, hours, or days of frustration and aggravation, I realize that not only have I not been taking care of myself, I've also been too wrapped up in everything that is going wrong. The minute I realize this, I remember how much church feeds me, friends feed me, and volunteer work feeds me, and I am in a much better position to balance things out without overwhelming myself. Taking care of your spirit can involve religious worship, exploring your talents, or anything that puts you more in touch with your emotions or true self. Nurturing your body and mind allows your spirit to thrive.

Spirit is the tie that pulls everything together. Because so many of us are lost in thoughts about what people see on the outside, our feelings have become secondary. And if we are not listening to our deepest feelings — our concerns and our joys — we are not able to become all that we were created to be. Spirit generates excitement, joy, curiosity, and the appreciation of beauty in everyday life, including your own beauty. If we can begin to pull off the layers that our spirit is buried under, bit by bit we will uncover an intriguing individual. Each time you tell yourself you are worthy, a layer comes off. Each time you take a risk and try something new, a layer comes off. Each time you take the time to read a story to your child, another layer comes off. Closer and closer that spirit comes to the surface, ready and willing to take you to undiscovered territory. This process can be exciting and even a bit frightening, but it is more than worth it. Your spirit is there, whether you know it or not. Now is the time to uncover it, slowly, patiently, and joyously.

Wouldn't it be great if you finish reading this book only to find that all the aspects of your life — physical, mental, and spiritual — have become perfectly balanced? Let's pause here and remember that this book is called *Reality Fitness* and that, therefore, reality is what I encourage. I would love nothing more than for you to instantly achieve balance, confidence, and a diet-free life. But the reality is you will have to work in stages to implement all that you've learned and to assess what does and doesn't work for you. I have written this book to help you visualize your possibilities. I can't make that happen instantly, I can only plant the seeds.

MY PERSONAL BALANCING ACT

To illustrate the process of change, I want to share more of my journey with you. Growing up, the idea of being content and at peace with myself was completely foreign to me. I first realized the need for balance during my first pregnancy, though I didn't know what I was seeking at the time. It was that realization that brought me to where I am now. Though I may not have fed myself positive messages as a young adult, and I certainly didn't respect the gift of my body, my spirit was much more powerful — as evidenced by my kindergarten report card that pointed out I talked too much but was full of spirit!

Throughout my life my spirit has enabled me to visualize and dream about all that was possible for me. My desire to help others while helping myself has made dreams come true for me. When I decided to get involved in personal training, people thought I was nuts, but my spirit didn't. When I wanted to write a book to further help other people, I heard from plenty of skeptics, but my spirit said, "Go for it!" My spirit has pushed me forward in times when I felt the only way to go was backward. As I trusted and grew with my spirit, I passed its messages to my mind, telling it that I could achieve anything I wanted to. As I began to excel and work toward my dreams and goals, suddenly my body began working for me, my healthy normal body that gave me the freedom to walk, run, skip, jump, and sing with joy. So part of my balance came through with accepting myself, trusting myself, and knowing that the only thing holding me back is me. I had no desire to sit back; I wanted to learn to make the best of all that was possible for me. Unfortunately, for a while dieting took my spirit and stifled it. It was getting off the diet and focusing on fitness that gradually brought me back to my center.

ONE MORE REASON NOT TO DIET

If we strive toward *our* idea of beauty, we will reduce our inner struggles over self-acceptance. If we believe we look great in the body we're in, we will find peace. If we strive to dress and act like the person we know ourselves to be, we will discover contentment. In any area of life, finding what feels right for you heightens your essence, because you are being true to yourself. My friends, it is time to "dis" the diet game and work toward true balance.

When it comes to dieting, begin with an understanding of what is and is not acceptable as far as lifestyle changes. Take a look at where you are right now. Are you a new mom? Are you working your way up the corporate ladder putting in sixty-to-seventy-hour weeks? Are you a grandmother taking care of an ailing partner or making visits to a nursing home? All these factors come into play when you're seeking balance. You must cut yourself some slack and be realistic. Starting a diet under any of these circumstances would be counterproductive. Balance is achieved through making positive choices that are most congruent with your life. And generally speaking, a diet boasting of a weight loss of thirty pounds in thirty days, for example, is not congruent with attaining anything healthy!

When I stopped spending my valuable time on nutty diet programs, I slowly began to discover more about me as a person, more about what I really liked and didn't like, more about what was possible. I wasted so much energy during the years I dieted, focusing my time on little else. In other words, there was absolutely no balance in my life during my dieting fixation. I am asking you now to please throw away your "miracle diet" accessories and begin doing good things for yourself. The twentieth century is going to be known as the century of diets. Wouldn't it be wonderful to move into the new millennium as liberated women no longer bound by the ties of the diet industry?

JOURNAL TO BALANCE

Open your journal to the next empty page. At the top, print in bold letters *I am most happy when*...and leave about ten lines underneath. Then write another heading that says, *I find I have the most difficulty with*.... Continue on to next page as needed and start another heading, *What I have wanted to do my whole life is*...again leaving about ten spaces. Your final heading should be *My special gifts and talents are*....

I encourage you to think long and hard about this

exercise. Don't expect yourself to do this in one evening; it will more than likely take a week or even a month. As you discover what centers you, you will be able to respond at greater length and with more ease and honesty. Balance begins to appear when you start following through with things you enjoy and that enhance your life. Look deep inside yourself to discover what gives you purpose and brings you joy. This can be a very difficult thing to do, so take your time and think about it while you walk, run, bike, or swim. As you make your lists, really listen internally. How do you feel as you write these words down? Do the words feel right or not? Or are you writing what you think you should write? When you really listen to yourself, you can gain some pretty incredible insights about exactly what you need.

BRINGING MIND, BODY, AND SPIRIT TOGETHER

Fitness is synonymous with a good balance of mental, physical, and spiritual health. So exercising your muscles, feeding yourself good things, thinking positive thoughts, and volunteering at the soup kitchen all go a long way toward making you feel like your life is in sync. Be open to all the things that make you uniquely you, accept them, and, for goodness sake, move on. By getting over the fact that my parents weren't perfect (because I discovered that neither was I) I was able to embrace my own imperfections (or perceived imperfections) and understand what makes me tick. Think of accepting yourself and where you are as unloading extra weight and bringing your personal scale into a state of balance — a more fulfilling way of losing "extra weight" than dieting!

And remember, balance cannot be attained overnight. Discovering who you are is an ongoing process that unfolds like a blooming flower if we don't force the petals open. There will be times when you close up, but you will open again when the time is right. Sometimes the road will seem very long; sometimes you'll reach a fork and experience uncertainty. Exercise can be intimidating — am I doing too much or not enough? We'll explore that so you are able to answer those questions for yourself and do what is right for you. Accept that life is a labyrinth and enjoy the unique experience of learning the paths that will ultimately lead you closer to the healthy life you so richly deserve.

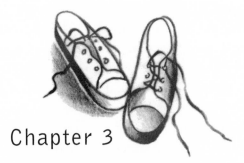

Chapter 3

DISCOVERING WHAT MOVES YOU!

Exercise is to the body
what books are to the mind

During the last twenty-five years, exercise has gone through some pretty interesting changes. Women have gone from hanging laundry as their only form of exercise to doing three thousand leg lifts a day to rid themselves of their "unsightly thighs." In this chapter we'll explore how structured exercise programs have evolved and help you discover practical exercises to assist you on your journey to balancing exercise.

Remember "Feel the Burn!" and "No Pain, No Gain"? I can still picture Jane Fonda, with those leg warmers hugging her long, lean thighs. Her intentions were great — she wanted to get more women exercising — though misconstrued. Jane's videos encouraged movement along with obsession, and women striving to attain Jane's perfectly sculpted body were coming up short. Her videos went on to influence a whole run of videos featuring "fitness beauties" promising flatter tummies and thinner thighs. We can be grateful that Jane raised the general level of awareness about exercise. But women had access to little that would enlighten them about the correlation between good health and exercise, and Jane's videos shared little information about overall health and wellness or reality.

In the 1980s, when the video craze was beginning, exercise was seen only as the ticket to having a great body. As exercise videos grew in popularity, so did our focus on weight and size. Every exercise video "hostess" had a great body and unending energy. We all wanted to possess that energy and body, so we kept buying the videos in hopes that maybe just the right one would do the trick. I remember renting one of those videos in my early twenties and watching this buff babe jump up and down with *nothing* on her body moving. How real is that? The truth was that reality didn't even enter the equation, and, after all, they were trying to sell videos! All I know is that it worked on me, as it did on so many other women. I wanted a body just like those I saw on

TV, and that's exactly where the trouble begins. I know that at one time I believed if I purchased the right exercise tape, I would look just like the model on the cover. Much to my disappointment, I still jiggled when I jumped. So I would continue my search for yet another program that would make me "perfect." In the 1980s, aerobics was hot. Women filled church halls and gyms jumping around in their leotards in an effort to become thin. For some it worked, but for others, injury after injury prevented them from continuing. Others, who weren't getting the results they wanted, simply quit.

In the early 1990s, the leg warmers vanished, and Jane Fonda went from "Feel the Burn" to "Ease the Burn" through yoga. She exchanged jumping for mantras. But because of Jane's trailblazing, everyone who ever exercised in their life (or who had claimed to) became part of the exercise video scene, and sales in exercise videos skyrocketed, from the FIRM to Richard Simmons to Susan Powter. Though Jane ditched the leg warmers for leggings and lost the feel-the-burn approach, her yoga tapes still weren't educating women about balanced living. In other words, videos were still presenting mixed messages and poor information. Cindy Crawford came out with a video that put women in traction, and soon anyone who looked decent in a leotard was coming out with an exercise video.

Unfortunately, those buying these videos didn't

have a clue about what was safe and appropriate for them, and not all the instructors were well qualified to teach exercise. Susan Powter's message of "just move" was probably the closest to reasonable and did get some sedentary individuals to simply move their bodies. As the 1990s came to a close, Jane Fonda continued to focus on balance, Cindy Crawford came out with an "improved" video, using safer technique with the guidance of a personal trainer, and Susan Powter disappeared from sight. And most of us, myself included, did not end up with Cindy Crawford bodies, just a nice collection of videotapes gathering dust on some remote part of our bookshelves. This is not to say that these exercise videos didn't have their effect. Between those videos and the increasingly popular diet programs, the foundation was being laid for a generation obsessed with their bodies, with no change in sight.

I ditched the videos as yet another failed attempt in the weight loss sport and sought out yet another strategy in hopes of slimming success. Some of my friends were taking aerobics classes so I thought I'd give it a try. I didn't know what to expect when I signed up for my first class and it's a good thing, I would have never followed through with it! Little did I know that I would become the poster child for exercise fashion faux pas! Everyone there was in matching leotard sets, and I walked in wearing my "I Love the Jackson 5" T-shirt and gray sweatpants with grass-stained sneakers. I felt like I was crashing a sorority party! Then, to add to my comfort level, some woman (a charter member of the aerobics police) pointed out that I was standing in a reserved spot. She made it clear that the spot was reserved for a "regular," and I was clearly an "irregular."

I complied (embarrassment and anger building inside) and moved to the back of the room thinking, "Why am I here?" Then the instructor, another member of the aerobic police, lost no time in informing me that if I was having difficulty keeping up (since it was my first class), maybe I'd be more comfortable just watching. At that point, exercise seemed pretty uninviting, and I left the class vowing to never go through an experience like that again. My story is not unique; many people have felt embarrassed, unwelcome, and awkward in various exercise classes. Unfortunate experiences like mine can ruin exercise, maybe even permanently, for the people who would benefit most from learning to use their bodies in a supportive environment.

WHERE ARE WE NOW?

Currently only 22 percent of Americans are regularly active, meaning they perform thirty minutes of moderate exercise most days of the week, as recommended by the College of Sports Medicine. Additionally, according to the National Health and Nutrition Examination Survey

(NHANES), obesity in children is up a remarkable 56 percent — the result of chronic inactivity. Our nation as a whole is out of shape, with the number of inactive people growing every day. Sadly, most of us (especially those us who have gone to sadistic exercise classes!) think that exercise is just a lot of blood, sweat, and tears. Women in particular tend to equate exercise with punishment, that is, punishment for having an imperfect body. "Because I am overweight and less than perfect, I must force myself into some rigid exercise program," or so the thinking goes. And rather than fight the all or nothing idea of exercise, we remain uneducated about what exercise options are available to us.

We are finally learning more from medical professionals about the long-term benefits, both physical and mental, of exercise. We know that if we exercise as frequently as possible, without killing ourselves or causing ourselves pain, we can help to prevent diseases such as diabetes — recent research shows exercise to be more important than anything else in preventing it — as well as hypertension, obesity, and a list of other ailments connected to an inactive lifestyle. Yet so many people still go to great lengths to avoid it. The reasons for this are myriad. On top of equating exercise with punishment, we also equate it with having a perfect body. And since everyone knows they can never have a perfect body, why bother exercising? In addition, many people feel that exercise requires more time than they have, or they've had similar experiences to my aerobics class nightmare and after that, who'd want to exercise? And let's not forget the all-too-common scenario of expending all your energy at the gym trying to figure out how some machine works with no one around to help you. Most often the comments I hear from my clients about exercise are of doom and gloom, and that's unfortunate.

Today the choices we have for exercise can be overwhelming. When I started exercising our choices were outside activities or aerobics classes or tapes. Now we have military classes, group step classes, kick-boxing classes, power yoga, water aerobics, and the list goes on. How do you determine where you'll feel comfortable and what program will be right for you? To help you along on your fitness adventure, I suggest hiring a personal trainer who will work with you one on one, assisting you with activities that are safe and appropriate for your fitness level. I'll provide more information on this option later in the chapter. Even with all these things to choose from, there are still barriers for those who are truly seeking a more active lifestyle. Many of these activities take place in the open area of clubs, which inexperienced exercisers find intimidating. Additionally, many daunting health club environments turn off those seeking a "gentle" entrance to the world of exercise.

Without improving their sensitivity, health clubs will continue to turn away the exact people they need to attract — those seeking a friendly, nurturing exercise environment. Take the time to explore different avenues until you find what is just right for you!

EXERCISE IS FOR EVERYONE

Okay, once you've found a comfortable exercise program, how do you keep consistent? I cannot say it often enough: It's imperative for you to find exactly what works for you and your lifestyle. The upside to the exercise tape explosion is increased options for those with little time, limited budgets, and the restrictions of having small children at home. The downside, of course, is that much of the exercise instruction is intimidating and vague, leaving the viewer feeling uncoordinated, unworthy, and ultimately unsuccessful. And because too many women expected to look like the models on the tape covers, after three weeks with little results, it was so long exercise, hello couch. Many women are under the impression that if they just spent three hours at the gym instead of one, they would attain the perfect body. If they just pushed themselves to the point of nausea, that tummy might get flatter.

One of the reasons I wanted to teach exercise was because I wanted to do so using nontraditional methods. That is, I refuse to go on and on about what great shape

I am in because of my exercise regime; rather, I explain my challenging journey to fitness and tell stories I think my clients can relate to. One of my clients was finding it particularly difficult to find time after work to exercise and she definitely did not want to get up at five in the morning. I told her how I used to put my walking shoes on before dinner so I would be mentally prepared after dinner to go for my walk. It worked for me and it ultimately worked for my client. We all know how hard it is to change our habits. And our habits — from bingeing or starving to running twenty miles or doing nothing — do need changing. We need to find the middle ground; without it, we'll be overwhelmed or under-challenged.

I also wanted to get my message out to the younger generation, the ones who most need to counterbalance all those hours of Nintendo and cable TV. In gym classes, the less coordinated kids are still picked last while the "natural" athletes are chosen first. The fact that I was never picked first or encouraged even when I knew I was doing my best definitely kept me out of the exercise arena. Why stay active when you feel you have no ability and are given little if any encouragement to be active? That's exactly how kids start out thinking.

We've got to turn around the way we look at exercise. I am no better than anyone else because I'm an exercise enthusiast. I've experienced exercise at its worst and its best, and I am therefore able to say with full confidence that exercise is meant for everyone. No one should have any reason to exempt him- or herself from daily movement — no one. It's simply finding what works for you. I was trained to help people discover and maintain a dedication to exercise and to live more health-conscious lives. If I make exercise an elitist activity, I am not following through on what I was trained to do. My ultimate goal is to encourage you to make exercise a natural part of your daily ritual, much like brushing your teeth. Exercise can be fun — really. It doesn't have to mean dressing up in skintight leotards and moving around like a Mexican jumping bean. Exercise can be a very personal, fulfilling experience.

EXERCISE BRINGS HARMONY

In Webster's New Collegiate Dictionary, the word *exercise* is defined this way: "To use repeatedly in order to strengthen or develop; bodily exertion for the sake of developing and maintaining physical fitness." Let's break down physical fitness to a more refined definition. Physical: "relating to the body" and fitness: "a suitable state, proper, harmony." Putting this all together, we can better understand the true definition of exercise: "a repeated movement of the body that brings about suitable harmony within oneself." Doesn't that sound great? Far more so than the definition most of us have ingrained, which is "really hard work that will bring on pain and sweat." Exercise should be viewed as a divine opportunity to enhance your mental, physical, and spiritual self. Additionally, it is equally important to understand the number of options available to you, no matter where you're starting. I am pleased to announce that you are no longer bound by the limits that ESPN and Ironman athletes have set forth. Exercise is not about four hours a day, seven days a week at the gym. If that were the case I'd be poo-pooing exercise right along with you. But the fact of the matter is that exercise is about moving your body in a way that works for you so that you can become healthier and stronger and enjoy it enough to stay with it forever!

There is a plethora of books out there with exercise routines advanced enough to challenge the Navy Seals. Unfortunately, many of us have bought a book, with a model on the cover, promising a complete body metamorphosis in six weeks. And as we now recognize, any major transformation in six weeks is impossible. Exercise is never finished in six weeks. Knowing that, there may be an aspect of the exercise program that you do like. Take the pieces that you do like and begin there. Just because a book tells you to do this program every day so that you can be a knockout doesn't mean you should.

During my years as a fitness trainer, I have seen many women who didn't exercise because nothing they did made a difference. But picture this: A sixty-year-old woman who has never exercised in her life takes a t'ai chi class, and it literally changes her life. She becomes more agile and less likely to incur injury, and her self-esteem improves greatly. Or a fifty-year-old woman bound by endless diets and disastrous exercise regimes completes a century bike ride after discovering (finally) an activity she adores. Or the forty-year-old woman who was never particularly athletic but manages to train for and complete her first marathon. How about the thirty-year-old woman who picks up jazz dance classes again, which give her more confidence and fun than anything she's done in years? These women have broken with tradition, meaning they've explored exercise options that appealed to them and have enjoyed and maintained a consistent exercise regime. Had they limited their exercise options, they would have been limiting their potential to have a healthy life. Are you the same?

MOVEMENT IS MOVEMENT IS MOVEMENT

Take a look at how much our modern lifestyle has "downsized" our physical activity. In the 1950s, 1960s, and 1970s, we were still getting up to change the channels, we were hanging laundry out to dry, we were walking more, and computers were simply not a part of our everyday life. Making things from scratch created even more physical activity. My grandmother used to tell me,

"Exercise is a fad. We never had to dress up and go to exercise classes. Go outside and play, for heaven's sake!" She was raised on a farm and started working a factory job at twelve years old. Her exercise came naturally through intense *daily* physical activity. To my grandmother, the idea of dressing up in a skimpy leotard to exercise was nuts, and she was on to something. In fact, I think another reason people don't exercise is that they don't want to be seen in public sweating and appearing awkward. They're also worried about having the appropriate exercise gear. Forget regulation. It's far more important to be comfortable than fashion conscious. Be comfortable during exercise; all you need are a comfy pair of sweats or shorts with a T-shirt and strong, supportive shoes. Jeans and a T-shirt and comfy sneakers on a beautiful fall day provide all you need for a satisfying walk.

The bottom line is that exercise isn't a fad; it's a must. Our lifestyles no longer provide us with the necessary physical activity we need to stay strong and healthy. As I stated earlier, our country is leading the way in obesity. We need to give our children as well as ourselves the opportunity to overcome an inactive lifestyle. Exercise, moving our bodies, is what will keep us all healthy and enjoying life more fully. It's unfortunate that so many of us think exercise means all or nothing. Movement is movement is movement is movement, period. The message I want to repeat until I'm blue in the face is that each of our bodies have different needs, and no one exercise program is right for everyone. It all comes down to finding what is right for you and your incredible body.

Our bodies are absolutely extraordinary in their abilities. Down to the finest detail, they were designed to move. Why then do we turn something as natural as exercise into something unnatural? We've got to sneak it in to our lives in small increments. How many times during the course of a day, a week, or month do you stop and thank your body for what it enables you to do, whether it's walking up and down the stairs, strolling through the park, or carrying a child?

Think about what you do in a day and how much time you end up sitting rather than standing. Most of my clients with young kids tell me, "Oh, but I'm running all day long! I'm taking them to soccer games, basketball practice, track meets." Well, it's great that you're so reliable and the kids get where they need to be, but the fact is you're not carrying them on your back to get them there. Instead, you are sitting on your bum driving them around. That doesn't do much for your cardiovascular health.

It is a unanimous opinion among my clientele that when they exercise they feel better. There's yet to be a time when a client has come into the studio feeling lousy (mentally or physically) that she doesn't leave feeling at least 75 percent better. Exercise is a natural mood elevator. Without getting too technical, exercise triggers endorphins in your mind that create a "feel good" sensation in your body. Exercise is a natural "health elevator." You are doing so many wonderful things for yourself when you walk or exercise. Imagine if Monet or Renoir had never been allowed to draw or paint. Their talent may have withered away and died. That is just what happens to our bodies when they are not given the opportunity to do what they were created to do: move. Your body needs exercise to thrive, to feed itself, to be all that it was intended to be. So if you can't get your body moving because you have a bad history with exercise, rethink your position and offer your body exercises the way you might offer a good friend consolation during a difficult time.

A potential client came into my studio eight weeks before her son was to be married. She was feeling lethargic and "old" and wanted to look and feel better before the wedding. Fortunately, she understood that no miracles would happen to her body in eight weeks, but she thought she might be able to make some modest improvements in herself. Her first positive step was not setting unrealistic expectations about beginning an exercise program. Instead, she dedicated herself to improving her overall health. Her dedication paid off.

After eight weeks of commitment to her exercise program, her doctor reduced her arthritis medication, she went down a dress size, and she felt better than she had in years. She had never even thought about the exercise having an effect on her arthritis, and even her physician was impressed with the results!

I am not exaggerating when I say that exercise can enhance your life in ways you may have never even thought about. Exercise is about giving and receiving. If you give your body all the exercise and good nutrition it needs, you will in turn receive a better quality of life. There is a catch, however: You must really want the best for yourself simply because you deserve it.

EXERCISE IS FOREVER

In my studio I use wipe boards to post motivational thoughts and weekly suggestions for exercise. One day my daughter came to work with me and asked if she could write the words for the week. My first thought was no, it wouldn't look professional and clients might not be able to read it. But she pleaded, and I agreed. To my surprise her words expressed my whole philosophy about exercise. The board read as follows: "It's exercise time, make it fun. Run around the block with your neighbor. Get your neighbor to run with you in the yard real fast. Play baseball, basketball, tennis, or how about capture the flag? Don't be lazy, be moveable. What are the three laziest things? Sitting, watching TV, and playing Nintendo."

From the mouths of babes. My clients loved her words. They agreed that we need to be "moveable" and to have more fun. Most important is that the message of being active doesn't differentiate between the twenty-year-old and the seventy-five-year-old. Movement is for every body!

Exercise begins where you feel most comfortable starting. If you want to use my suggestion above and hire a trainer, great! If not, I believe the best place to begin is to envision the type of exercise you would like to do and of how it might feel. Let's say you've always wanted to take a dance class. What type of dance? How would it feel when you begin to dance? Even if you're like me and your spouse refuses to budge on the dance floor, don't give up. Dance classes provide many options. In college I got involved in theater and was often in the ensemble that provided the choreography. I had never taken dance before that, but dance and I connected, and I was hooked. I ended up directing some choreography routines, and after a couple of years I felt I had found my "sport."

That's the point: You've got to feel good doing what you're doing so that you'll want to continue with it. But you don't have to stop with one activity! Generally, when my clients start a new activity, it gives them the confidence they need to explore other areas. One of my clients only enjoyed the stationary bike for five minutes at a time. She used it throughout the winter and when spring came she asked for a real bike. By Christmas the next year she had ridden more than one thousand miles and decided her goal for the next spring would be to enter a race. She did and finished it! Some may not take it that far, but you can start off with a simple walk around the block, turn that block into two blocks, and after that consider adding some hills.

Once you realize how much you can do, and make it happen, you'll understand the importance of moving forward with new and exciting challenges. Most important is to pay attention to how great you feel when you meet the challenges you've set. Whatever you choose to do, keep in mind that you will have strong exercise weeks and slower ones. Some days I exercise, other days I don't. It's not the end of the world; I just make sure I add a little more time my next session. What's important is your desire to become stronger, healthier, and more "moveable."

JOURNAL TO SUCCESS

Okay, let the fun begin! Take out your journal and think about what you enjoyed doing when you were younger. If you're currently inactive, also known as being in "slug mode," think about an activity you have considered but never pursued. It can be anything from rock climbing to badminton, from golf to tennis (there are lessons for beginners), from *tai kwon do* to ballet. Your options are endless. Make a list of anything that sparks your enthusiasm. Try not to think of exercise strictly in terms of regimented programs. Orienteering, hiking, kayaking, and roller-blading are just some of the possibilities. After you've listed some activities that sound fun and exciting, narrow them down to what is realistic for you. For example, I live in the Midwest, so learning to surf is going to be tough. I'm not saying I couldn't do it, but the likelihood of doing it consistently is impossible. However, I could come up with some other water activities that would be more suitable for this climate and available at the local YWCA. Then circle the activities that seem most suitable.

If you've circled your activities and are thinking, "Right, I have no time for any of this," stop right there. Remind yourself that each movement is a step forward. Take baby steps. Here's an analogy: As soon as a baby is born, does she immediately begin to walk? Of course not. She goes from being a blob to rolling over to pushing up to crawling to holding herself up and finally to putting one foot in front of the other. A child has no expectations, just the curiosity and excitement to forge ahead! In other words, you've got to start small with no expectations, just hope. Maybe your dream activity isn't "doable" right now. So figure out what is and start there. If you love to dance but can't make it to a class, there are videotapes out there that are fun to work with. If you've got small kids, put on some CDs and go nuts! If you love ballet but feel you're too out of shape, start with a yoga class to develop your flexibility. You can't change in a day what took years to develop. Inactivity didn't just happen over a long weekend; it gradually crept up over weeks, months, and years. If you look at the big picture, it can be too overwhelming. Just look at what is in front of you right now, and begin small and slow.

NOW WHAT?

Pick just one of the activities you circled. If that activity is walking, then that is where you need to start. Even five minutes a day walking around your block is a reasonable starting point for you. When my kids were babies, I used to put them in a Snuggli™ while I mowed the lawn, just so I could get some exercise while also keeping an eye on them. You've got to start somewhere. There has been much controversy over how much exercise is enough. Some experts push an hour a day, while others suggest thirty minutes most days for optimum benefits. I personally believe that forty-five minutes a day is ideal. Well, having a house on Maui is ideal but not practical for everyone, so do what is practical for you right now.

Your next step is to make a list of your exercise goals. Then decide what things you can reasonably do in a day to meet these goals. (It might also be a good idea to read the goal-setting chapter before you start.) Remember to evaluate whether these activities are realistic for you; it they're not, they're not going to work. Then you'll be ready to move ahead. Here's an example:

Activities I Like:
Dance (jazz, tap), walking, bike riding, tennis

What I Can Do:
Take an adult dance class once a week
Walk with my neighbor two times a week in the
    park
Sign up for tennis lessons
Use my treadmill or stationary bike three times a
    week for fifteen minutes

I highly recommend getting a physical before starting any new exercise program, even if you're starting with walking. You need a baseline to start from. If you decide to use a personal trainer, get a name from someone who has had experience with a trainer or interview a number of trainers before you settle on one. Make sure they're properly certified and have some experience, and most important, ask them about their philosophy regarding exercise. If she or he is rigid in her or his beliefs, than you need to find someone who shares your feelings and attitude about exercise. Think of selecting a trainer as you would choose a doctor. Take the time to choose carefully.

Personal trainers are not just to "pump you up"; they are there to guide you and support you through steps in determining which path to good health is right for you. They are there to teach you safe, practical exercise programs so that you'll be able to exercise for the rest of your life knowing what is safe, effective, and time efficient. Not all trainers are expensive, and a good one is worth every penny you spend. Not only will you garner needed tools for successful exercise programs but you will also have a cheerleader! Yes, I'm a little biased, but I feel strongly that hiring a trainer is the best money you can spend. Too many women begin an exercise program without a clue about what exercises and approach are best for their body type and lifestyle. I ask those unsure about hiring a trainer, "What would you rather spend your money on, medication for high blood pressure or a few sessions with a personal trainer?" And that's the bottom line, your health.

So what's the right amount of exercise? It's what works for you right now. Whatever it is, if you find it's too much, start off slower. No one (including me) said that going from being inactive to active would be easy.

But it will be much easier if you take the time to explore your options, your passions, and your true goals. Whichever route you choose, whether it's hiring a trainer or discovery through journaling, here are some valid reasons to begin an exercise program. Choose the reasons that resonate with you and write them in your journal next to your exercise choices. The reasons you choose will be the reasons you become more and more active and increase the quality of your health and life.

  a. To lower blood pressure and cholesterol and improve carbohydrate metabolism
  b. To increase self-esteem through enhanced coordination
  c. To preserve the body's muscle
  d. To increase metabolism
  e. To improve confidence that helps reduce stress
  f. To keep your weight at more of a consistent, healthful range than what's possible through dieting

I could list many more, but the bottom line is that exercise will enhance the quality of your life. I hope that the information I've shared has lightened a heavy load of fear or guilt or just plain inertia and put exercise into a more desirable light. I've said it before and I'll say it again: any amount of exercise is better than nothing. It's wonderful to see women start off with only five minutes of exercise a day and then within six months sign up for a three-mile walkathon for charity. Exercise will make you feel younger, stronger, and great all over. It can change the way you treat life and how life treats you! I invite you to take on the challenge of changing your life. So, where do you begin? At the beginning — let's go!

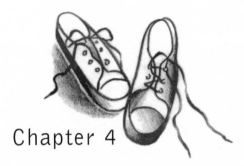

Chapter 4

SIMPLE SUGGESTIONS FOR GOOD NUTRITION

Diets allow us little food, little comfort, with little learned

In my diet and exercise experience, bringing good nutrition and exercise together was the biggest challenge. It seemed I could only focus on one or the other; I couldn't balance the two. I soon realized that I was trying to change too much at once. For instance, I would start walking every day and, at the same time, try to drastically change my eating habits. I would become frustrated within a week because I couldn't stick with it.

I've seen many diet and exercise failures caused by trying to change an entire life in a week. It's simply not possible. I've explained the importance of baby steps with exercise, and the same applies to nutritional changes. In this chapter, I'll discuss ways you can change your nutrition without forfeiting taste, as well as appreciating the impact whole foods have on your body. It's also important to learn the harmful effects chronic dieting has on your overall health. When we look at the traditional weight loss programs, food becomes the enemy. Reality Fitness is about building a positive relationship with food. Reality Fitness is about respecting your body enough to provide it with quality food. Reality Fitness uses food as a source of energy rather than a source of punishment.

HEALTHY FOOD FOR A HEALTHY BODY

It seems the majority of women were raised to be the purveyors of food, taking charge of everyone's nutritional quotient except their own. As a result, we continue to adapt our shopping and eating habits to accommodate busy schedules and changing diet fads. With every diet comes new foods, regardless of whether they're good for us or not. Perhaps we choose foods that are low fat, fat free, high carbohydrate, low carbohydrate, light, or, too often, fast. Some of these foods promise health benefits while others promise simply to help us with the battle of the bulge. Every week we hear about how these new "miracle" foods will lower our cholesterol, curb our appetite, or satisfy our sweet tooth with half the calories! Unfortunately, we are not educated about the ramifications of these processed, high-sugar foods. And, just as unfortunately, we aren't educated about the benefits of whole foods that make our bodies strong and healthy and, yes, even lean.

While we used to eat for nourishment, today convenience seems most important, regardless of how good the food is for our bodies. The busier our lives become the less we pay attention to the quality of food. Now we seek convenience and quantity, with pre-packaged and fast foods. Along with all of this food, our increasingly convenient lifestyles have become much less active. I truly believe that the accessibility of food, anytime, anywhere, has led to the demise of our country's nutritional habits. Generally speaking, most of us do not discern between nutritious food and junk food. We are eating processed fruit snacks instead of the fruits of the earth. The overconsumption of fat-free foods — fat-free does not mean calorie-free — and the overeating of processed, fast foods are two primary reasons for our country's obesity and disease problems.

Food is fuel for our bodies. Just as poor quality, leaded gas would ruin our cars, "junk food" can ruin our bodies. Without "premium" food, we will not function at our best. Eating well doesn't mean you have to eat enough for an army or that you eat two bites and then pronounce how full you are. Eating high-quality food (meaning fruits, vegetables, and whole grains) in reasonable amounts is one of the best things you can do to keep yourself healthy and strong.

Many things need to change regarding nutrition in this country, and how we view food is one of them. I deal with people every day who are struggling to understand their personal battles with food. Part of the problem is the power we've given to it. We've given it a life of its own, and it governs us from morning to night, especially those of us with children. With kids it often becomes all you think about, because of your responsibility to provide breakfast, snacks, lunch, more snacks, and then the evening meal. It's food, food, food!

Food often becomes an all-or-nothing proposition — much like exercise. We've taken what was meant to be a necessary, healthy staple of life and created a dysfunctional relationship! I believe that we must begin with the understanding that food doesn't make or break us. In other words, if we eat a piece of candy, we're not bad; if we opt for dessert, we are not undisciplined — though we do need to discern between overindulgence and periodic treats. We need to stop letting food define our mood and our sense of self-worth. Food is there to feed and nurture the body, not to torture it.

Food has become our enemy, but we need it to become our ally. You know how you feel when you eat well — more fresh veggies and fruit, less alcohol, and less sugar. It means fueling your body to the point of satisfaction, not to the point of feeling bloated. Maybe we don't know anymore what simply being satisfied feels like. It's not too much nor too little, it's just right. Take time to find what's just right for you.

A HEALTHFUL DIET VERSUS THE DIET OF THE MONTH

The word *diet* simply defines the food we ingest each day. But now it has become a four-letter word or a badge of honor, sometimes even a badge of martyrdom. Dieting has become a national pastime, with everyone waiting in line for the next diet of the month, guaranteed to make us all fit and trim.

There are some very valid diets out there: diets for diabetics, for stroke victims, for ulcer patients, and so forth. These are specific diets for specific needs. But I'm talking about the kinds of diets that offer you a perfect life if you only eat in a prescribed way. Unfortunately, when one diet doesn't come through for us, we're off to the next, and the cycle continues. But each time you toy with yet another diet, you are putting your health at risk mentally, physically, and emotionally. We have developed such a skewed view of food and diets that we don't know whether we're coming or going, losing or gaining, failing or succeeding.

Remember our new paradigms for the words *fat* and

weight from the introduction? Well, we also need to create a new paradigm for the word *diet. Diet* is actually a good word; it's diet*ing* that starts the trouble. As I stated above, *diet* means the food we consume that fuels our bodies, while *dieting* (and this is my personal definition) offers only the two d's: deprivation and depression. Though diet is rarely defined as dangerously low caloric intake, our current diet paradigm means self-inflicted starvation and deprivation through rigid programs allowing minimal food. Our old paradigm has made life very difficult for those of us who do not resemble runway models; we think that if we just starve ourselves, we can achieve that "perfect" body. Well, you know and I know that any nutrition program that provides dangerously low daily caloric allotments is unsafe and unrealistic. So how do we bring the word *diet* back to its original meaning?

Simply viewing diet as the fuel we give our bodies may spark a shift in the paradigm. To return to the gasoline analogy, the better grade of fuel we put in our bodies, the better our bodies will run. Your "regular" fuel is sweets, dairy, and fats. Your "unleaded" fuel is carbos and proteins. And your "premium" is fruits and veggies, fresh of course! And when we eat a healthful diet, we're not as prone to overeating. When you're aware of and concerned with what you're feeding yourself, you'll be aware of how much you actually need.

You see, a diet that consists of healthful eating is forever, while diets are a passing fancy that encourage unhealthy eating. Going on diet after diet takes a toll on your body and your mind. Understand that while we've created the difference between the words *diet* and *dieting*, in reality, they are one and the same. When you have a clear understanding of these words' true meaning, you will be able to stay on the road to healthy living and get off the diet-of-the-month club mailing.

JOURNAL TO GREAT NUTRITION

Study after study continues to show that those who keep track of their nutritional intake tend to eat better and to stay on a healthier nutrition program for longer periods. Many women panic when asked to keep track of what they eat because they become aware of how much "low-grade" fuel they're ingesting. Then they beat themselves up when they see the record of all the things they shouldn't be eating but are unable to make long-term changes. Many then try dieting to improve their food habits, but as we know, diets don't create long-term changes or habits. Why? See if any of these sound familiar: "Lose ten pounds in ten days, thirty pounds in thirty days, twenty inches in six weeks." And the list goes on. You cannot possibly make any long-term changes in ten, twenty, or thirty days. Permanent change takes time; it takes weeks, months, and even years.

Invariably when I ask a client to track her nutrition, the first words out of her mouth are, "Why? So you can see how bad I am?" The other common response is, "Do I have to tell the truth?" But the bottom line is, tracking what you eat is a wonderful way to see how your body responds to what you fuel it with. Yes, it also gauges how balanced your nutrition program is or isn't. But it's not an opportunity to beat yourself up; it's a chance to discover how to fuel yourself for good health. So let's start keeping track of what we eat and see what we learn.

I would encourage you to keep a separate journal for tracking your nutritional intake. A three-by-five note-book is perfect for keeping in your purse or backpack and taking along anywhere you go. Start as soon as you can, and write down everything that goes into your body —drinks, snacks, everything. How many times have you said, "Oh, I feel terrible. I know I overate today"? Well, by keeping track of what you eat, you may be able to pinpoint why you overdid it. Were you worried? Tired? Too busy? It might also help you see some patterns that you were unaware of. I once asked a client, who believed her only concern was a couple of coffees too many, to track her daily intake. When she did, she realized that she was drinking as many as sixteen cups a day! When I was training for the marathon, I wrote down everything I was eating so I could see what foods created more energy and what made me tired, gassy, and so on. Why not find out what fuel works best for you? You will never be able to change your current nutritional habits if you don't know where you are right now. And here's an added tip: Don't wait to record what you've been eating till the end of the day. Research shows that when you wait until evening to document your food intake, you may miss something. So after each meal and snack, jot it down. But it's not so much the calorie count I want you to focus on as it is the overall balance in your diet.

In addition to tracking your food intake, track how you feel after meals or after eating certain foods. You don't need to spend a huge amount of time on this. You can quickly jot down what you've eaten and then even create a system to designate your energy level that day. For example, HE equals high energy, LE equals low energy, PMS (well, we all know what that one is), and so on. You'll eventually begin to see a pattern in your energy levels, your cravings, and so forth. After you have tracked your nutrition for one week, I want you to look over it, carefully. As you do, circle with a red pen the eating habits you would like to change. It doesn't really matter how many things you circle, but be aware that trying to change everything overnight will just result in frustration and going back to old habits. I encourage you to focus on making changes one at a time. Doing so will help you to gradually change your habits and ensure long-term success. By success I mean fueling your body well consistently.

After you've circled all the things you'd like to change, pull out your journal. Skip a few pages from your last entry. At the top of a clean page write "Positive Changes for Positive Living." Beneath that, make a list of all the eating habits that you circled on your nutrition-tracking log. Now list in order of importance the changes you would like to make. Here's an example:

1. Eating late-night ice cream
2. Eating too much bread at evening meals
3. Eating my children's leftovers

After you have finished making your list, begin with the first item. Think of ways to change this habit gradually. For example, if you're currently eating ice cream every night, you can start by eliminating three ice creams a week, then four, then five, and so on. Remember, I do not encourage deprivation. Ice cream is fine — in moderation. Once you feel comfortable with your change, you can move on to the next one. Stick with a change until you have comfortably altered your habit. Even if it takes you six months to alter one habit, the important thing is that you are making permanent changes. If you take the time to methodically change a habit, you can bet that the change you make will be with you for the rest of your life.

Now go to the next clean page in your journal and make a heading out of the habit you are currently working on. Record your feelings about making this change. What is easy about making this change? What is challenging? Is it easier than you thought or is it a really hard habit to break? Closely tracking each change you're working on is a great way to work through the behavior you're trying to modify. Yes, this is basically behavior modification 101, but it works. You'll need plenty of room to write, so be sure to create a new page for each change you're working toward. Here is an example:

"LATE-NIGHT ICE CREAM"

June 25: Instead of ice cream I only had a yogurt. I still felt guilty, but I guess it's better than ice cream.

June 27: Decided to replace an old habit with a new one, so I bought a new book. Rather than eat ice cream, I've started reading. It's a little hard not to think about ice cream, but I feel better already not eating it late at night.

June 28: Went to a birthday party and had ice cream late, but I didn't have any cake, so I felt pretty good about that. I only had a small serving of the ice cream, and I didn't feel guilty — yay!

Again, let me remind you that you're not keeping this record to see what little discipline you have; rather, it's an opportunity to monitor your progress and to see where your greatest challenges lie. You don't have to write something in it every day, but if it's an everyday habit you're trying to break, it might be a good idea. Also, at the top right-hand corner of each page, write the word *diet*. Next to it, write your brief, revised, healthy definition so that you can begin to hold onto your new ideas about what it means to eat well. Now, instead of going *on* a diet, you are finding new ways to *alter* or *improve* your diet. Now you are seeking healthful eating instead of riding the wave of trendy diets.

A REALITY CHECK FOR HEALTHFUL EATING

Whenever a client tells me she has started a diet, the first question I ask is, "Is it realistic for you and is it something you can do for the rest of your life?" Generally, the response is, "I never thought of it that way. I just wanted to lose the weight." Remember: It is much better to aim for a healthy weight through reasonable nutrition than it is to starve yourself for six months. If you use the starvation approach, you know and I know you'll be back to where you started within a year. Learning to eat well consistently is a step toward taking control of your health, a preventative measure, a piece of the healthy-living puzzle. I don't have trouble blaming much of the poor eating habits of this country on the diet industry. We have come to accept that if we can't stick to a thousand-calorie-a-day diet, we have no self-discipline. But underfeeding ourselves has nothing to do with self-discipline and everything to do with false information — that is equating skinny with healthy. They're not the same thing!

For fifteen years I went from one diet to the next. Did I learn about eating well? No, but I certainly learned the precise caloric value in a chocolate bar and in potato chips! You *can* eat heathfully without counting calories, fat, or anything else. Eating well is about making choices that work best for your body. It doesn't take a genius to know that a fresh fruit salad is better for you than a candy bar. And you don't have to be a rocket scientist to know that a double cheeseburger is really more food than you need. Healthful eating means eating foods that make you feel good and that fit your lifestyle. Yes, sometimes fast food will fit into the equation, but do we really need a "biggie" to fuel our bodies adequately?

So many of us have dieted for years and are trying to figure out why none of the diets have worked. For too long we have practiced deprivation or excess and nothing in between. Reality Fitness is all about the in-between. Learning to eat well will take practice, research, and trial and error, and that's fine. We all overindulge at times, but it's not the end of the world. The problem is when overindulgence becomes the norm. Sure, there will be times when you'll splurge on a sundae or a wonderful piece of chocolate. That's okay! If you keep away from diets, no foods are off limits. What's important is that you learn what foods fuel you well for your day-to-day performance and what foods drag you down. You are now in a proactive position to make sound choices about your nutrition. Begin to experiment with new and exciting foods, plan meals, be creative. If you have children or a spouse, include them in making changes in your nutrition. We need to take the responsibility by selecting foods that strengthen and energize us and our loved ones.

Of course, most of us have spent our entire lives developing our nutritional habits, so don't expect to change them overnight. Also keep in mind that everyone's diet (and I mean it in the healthy sense of the word) is different. Commercial diets are usually one size fits all. How successful will anyone be on a generic program? If one client is a working mom and another is a stay-at-home mom, my nutrition suggestions are going to be much different because of the difference in daily schedules. And certainly holidays, seasonal changes, and stressful events all affect how we eat. That's one reason why you need to spend a good amount of time tracking nutrition and experimenting before you find just what works for you. Don't worry if you do overeat at Thanksgiving. It's not an everyday occurrence, and, also, if you don't deprive yourself, you'll be less inclined to overeat generally. Holidays are the time for celebration, so celebrate! It's when that celebration goes on for 365 days a year that you need to reevaluate.

It all goes back to the all-or-nothing syndrome. Eating well isn't about depriving yourself. It's about ridding yourself of the diet mentality and instead acquiring good information about fueling your body properly. When I realized that no diet in the world was going to make me a different person, I became far more interested in finding ways to make the most of who I am and what I have the potential to be. But it took time and introspection. When we begin to make changes, we rarely think about what obstacles lie ahead, and when we encounter them unprepared, we sometimes revert to our old habits. So do yourself a favor, and spend a full year making sure that the changes you've decided to make are realistic for you and your lifestyle. It's exciting to rid yourself of the diet mentality and finally understand that healthy eating no longer means *not* eating.

A PARENT'S GUIDE TO HEALTHFUL EATING

About ten years ago, after spending some serious time evaluating the foods I was eating, I began to take a look at my family's nutrition. Mind you, at that time my husband, Bill, was a true meat and potatoes man, so I was cooking mainly to please the palate, not the body. Rather than change everything overnight, I decided that I would sneak one heart-healthy meal in a week and see if he noticed. Heart healthy for my family meant adding more fruits and vegetables and eliminating fried foods, gravies, and salty foods. After a while, cooking heart-heathy meals became a game. Bill had to guess if the meal I made was heart healthy or not. He was certain that healthy foods tasted like cardboard and were limited to tofu and bean sprouts! It was a wonderful way to become creative with my cooking, but it also made the transition to better eating much easier for my family. Instead of frying meat for stew I would boil it first or grill it. Instead of making gravy (which my husband loves) I discovered I could make a healthier "gravy" from low-sodium bouillon, corn starch, and spices. Over time, especially if you're in charge of grocery shopping and food prep, you can sneak in more and more healthy options.

I learned to adopt better nutrition habits by again, taking baby steps. I started by reading *Cooking Light* magazine, which contained clear information and had recipes I could pronounce and ingredients that I could find at the grocery store. I discovered how interesting this kind of cooking could be. So often I hear, "All that low-fat food has no taste; it's bland!" When we are all so used to processed food, which is full of sodium and sugar, we have to adjust our palates to new tastes.

Cooking nutritious meals doesn't have to be complicated or bland. We tend to be creatures of habit, so it can be difficult to change years of established cooking habits. That's why I suggest you start out slowly with one meal a week, like I did. Or maybe one meal a month is more doable for you right now, and that's fine. Also, don't cook something you don't like! If you see a heart-healthy recipe for squid and you don't like squid, don't prepare it! Seek out recipes that include things you like and sound good to you. Read light cooking magazines, and even some fitness magazines, to find recipes for nutritious meals.

During the last ten years I have learned so much about cooking tasty and healthful foods. I feel good about the food I put on my table at night and the food I feed myself. Sure, there are still those fast-food days, but I can honestly say that I just don't have the stomach for fast food anymore. Though I was once the queen of fast food, I find that I have more energy and feel more balanced when I eat healthful foods.

Begin this week by exploring new recipes. Buy a three-ring binder and some plastic inserts. Each time you find a recipe you like and that you would prepare again, store it in your binder. After a year you'll have a personal cookbook with all the recipes you enjoy. It's a great way to discover your style of healthy eating and to pass it on to those you love! Changing how you feed yourself and your family doesn't happen overnight. It's a long process that involves a lot of experimenting and patience. There is no right or wrong here, only what works for you. What matters is that you are establishing habits and gaining knowledge that will carry you through the rest of your life. Have fun!

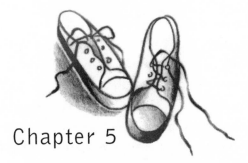

Chapter 5

SETTING REALISTIC GOALS

Make sure your goals are from the heart, for the heart's song reveals your true desire

Imagine not having to weigh in each week. No one's shaking a contemptuous finger at you because you didn't stick to your eight-hundred-calorie-a-day diet. Wouldn't it be great to find such a program? Well, you already have: It's called Reality Fitness, which is all about discovering an appropriate passage to becoming a happier, healthier, more productive you. It is about setting realistic goals for yourself so that your passage is successful.

Think about the goals you set for yourself each time you embarked on a new diet. Does fitting into a size four ring a bell? How about weighing exactly what you weighed in high school? Or exercising every day? We have all set goals like that. The problem with each of these goals is that they are not healthy, long-term, realistic goals. What will fitting into a size four do for your cholesterol level? Will weighing what you weighed in high school give you more energy? What about exercising every day? Do you see yourself sticking with that goal a year from now? Five years from now? Ten years from now?

Furthermore, do you really want to work toward these goals or are they goals you *think* you should be setting for yourself? I have yet to see a popular weight-loss plan that takes you beyond losing weight and provides steps for long-term healthy living. The only kudos that come from those rigid programs are when the scale displays the "perfect" numbers. But after you've lost the weight, you're on your own, baby. Imagine a nutrition program whose philosophy is, "We don't focus on the weight, we focus on you because your health and well-being come first."

What a refreshing approach that would be! No more blaming yourself because you've failed yet another program. No more shame incurred by a group weigh-in session. My years of trial and error and short-term successes with every diet and exercise program forced me to take a look at why and how: Why was I unable to "be disciplined for the rest of my life"? And how might I discover a program that assured long-term success without the fear of failing (again)? It slowly became clear to me that every diet and exercise program out there is generic. They assume that everyone can follow the program and be equally successful. That's like designing one shirt and one pair of pants in one size and color and expecting them to fit and appeal to everyone. That obviously wouldn't work, so why do we believe that the same diet would suit everyone? It won't, and that's precisely why you need a successful system to encourage long-term healthy living habits.

The goal-setting system that I developed as part of Reality Fitness will take you through the steps that I finally successfully followed after failing time and time again with the one hundred plus diets I tried. We fail when we don't have a clear understanding of our ultimate goal. Most diet goals — losing ten pounds by summer or having a twenty-six-inch waist again — may sound clear-cut, but in essence they reflect only a desire. And they have nothing to do with your overall health. As a twenty-year-old woman I started Weight Watchers™ mainly so that I could fit into my teenage jeans again. But I was fortunate, because it ended up teaching me how to eat well for the rest of my life. I lost more than forty pounds and learned about healthy balanced nutrition. There was no quick and easy, no guarantee — just a simple lesson in eating well.

So for more than twenty years I have retained much of what I learned then. Obviously, there was something in that program that worked for me and that complemented my lifestyle. Sure, I didn't follow the program at times, but I never felt like a failure, and I continued to learn. That's because although my initial goal had been to lose weight, it very soon became to continue learning how to take care of myself, and that was an attainable goal for me. I had discovered a program that worked for me, and that's exactly what realistic goal setting will do for you.

DIET FAILURE, GOAL-SETTING SUCCESS

Often when we embark on a quick-and-easy diet or exercise program, we rarely examine the long-term benefits. Why should we? We want twenty pounds off today! We push aside the hazards or limitations in favor of what really matters: being skinny. These diets all sound so good that it's hard to think that they won't work for you, especially with all those great guarantees of thinner thighs and flatter tummies. But the truth is that diets don't work for the long term, leaving us depressed, frustrated, and back to square one.

Every time I failed a diet, I would blame myself and feel hopeless. At first I never considered that maybe the program was unrealistic or inappropriate for my lifestyle. After I "failed" — that is I didn't become as thin as I had wanted — with each weight-loss program, I would be lured into another. I lost sight of my health because of my goal — really society's goal — of becoming thinner. Societal pressures had me convinced that if only I was thin enough, I would be happy, rich, and beautiful. But if you're setting a goal to accommodate someone else's agenda, it just ain't gonna happen! The truth is, a goal can never be attained if it isn't your very own. A goal has to be your true desire. Then, and only then, can you be passionate enough about it to make it happen. And you can!

SUCCESS THROUGH FAILURE

It may sound odd, but failure is the only way to reach success. Without some failures along the way, you cannot discover the right path. But because of its negative connotations, I don't even use the word *failure* in my studio, I use the word *experience*. Every diet I went through was an experience that taught me what doesn't work for me, and I kept trying until finally one day I said, wait a minute, something is not right. The more I diet the worse I feel, and the worse I feel the more I diet.

So how did I pull myself out of the chronic teeter-totter diet affliction? Basically, I had had enough. I was through beating myself up for something that I didn't understand or have control over. As I looked around at my friends and family, I saw more and more women who were losing the battle of diet and exercise. Their continued failure at diets and exercise regimes sucked away more and more of their self-esteem, leaving them feeling desperate. And the more desperate we become, the more likely we'll attempt anything (regardless of the ramifications) to achieve our unrealistic goals. Diets grab hold of us when we are most vulnerable. They prey on that vulnerability, and in the end, we shoulder the blame and move on to the next program. It was time for me to change all that.

I ultimately got off that teeter-totter by having a clear-cut vision of what I truly wanted to achieve. I realized that losing weight would not affect the core of who I really was, and I set about setting some realistic goals that were more about the overall quality of my life — feeling good physically and mentally. I am sure that if we had been schooled in setting practical goals before starting any of the hundreds of diet and exercise programs we've attempted, our failure rate would have been greatly reduced. When the goals you've set for a particular program do not jibe with your lifestyle, abilities, or real desires, you know that's a program to walk away from. Once I carefully considered what I really wanted for my health, I recognized how important realistic goal setting would be for long-term success.

SETTING REALISTIC GOALS

Do you look at New Year's resolutions as goals? Well, that's exactly what they are. Every year millions of people make resolutions that never make it past March 1 because they are goals that sound great at the time but are completely unrealistic. For example, resolving to lose thirty pounds in the next year has no basis in reality. In fact, it's something that you've wanted to do for the last ten years, and every year, after a month or so, you cast the goal aside because it's totally incongruent with your lifestyle and fitness level.

My resolution every year was to take up dance again. Every January I would tell myself that I was going to sign up for a dance class that met three times a week. I never seemed to factor in my full-time job, four kids, my writing, and so on. Why did I think my life could suddenly accommodate a three-day-a-week dance class? It just was not a realistic goal for me. Even though three days a week would be ideal, it wasn't practical, and I had other things at the top of my priority list. I obviously needed to figure out (if I truly wanted to do it) how to fit dance in. So I decided to try once a week, which was much more doable for me, and it worked. I did attend dance class faithfully every week until I was able to add more time. You see, there's much we may want, but we've got to put these desires in perspective and decide what will work for where we are right now. Take it in steps. Most important, set a goal that is for you and only you. Dancing three times a week might have been my desire, but it wasn't right for me. But a class once a week still gave me the great pleasure of dancing, and it fit my life.

As I've said before, I often tell my clients, "If you're starting an exercise or nutrition program, you need to ask yourself if it's something you can do for the rest of your life. If the answer is no, stop right now, reassess, and start over."

START SMALL

Goal setting was rarely discussed in my family, especially since my father didn't believe that women could succeed. It wasn't until I began working for a health club and was living on my own and destitute that I discovered setting goals. At that time I was (or so I was told) a phenomenal sales associate. After just six months with the company, I had the largest sales volume, and I was only seventeen. My boss was the first person who encouraged me to set goals so that I could generate more income. It was a revolutionary concept: to state your desire, set a plan, see if it fits your philosophy, and, *voilà*, success!

Every goal that I set at work, I reached. But at first, it was a challenge. Some goals sound stupid or impossible. But like anything new, the more you do it the easier it becomes. I remember when I first started setting goals I showed them to my boss and asked him, "Are these right?" He responded, "If they're right for you, then they're just right." His attitude had a lot to do with my success at the health club. It's been stated that those who set goals tend to be more successful in all areas of their lives. Goals help keep our direction clear and our motivation high.

Setting goals is the best way to get excited about possibilities, that is, if the goals reflect your true desires. Many of us know we want to lose weight, but that isn't a specific goal, it's too general. By getting in touch with what your true needs are you will be less likely to become involved with a program that is short-term, ineffectual, and ultimately dangerous. A rigid diet is not something you can do forever, so why even begin? Begin slowly by selecting a small goal. Stick with that for a while and see how it goes, then think about setting another goal. Being realistic as you set your goals encourages permanent lifestyle changes. When setting goals, ask yourself if they are conducive to your life and focused on your health. If the answer is "yes," then you're on the right track.

THE FIRST STEP: DISCOVERING WHAT YOU WANT

Since we are focusing on creating a healthier lifestyle for you, our emphasis will be on healthy lifestyle goals. Before you get started, we must uncover what your true goals are. How do you know if they reflect your true desires? It helps to ask yourself if you're willing to make some changes in order to reach your stated goal. Now is the time to think about what you *really* want. Think about what makes you smile, what makes you feel passionate, what propels you forward even when you're stressed. Don't ask someone else! Don't let your goals be your mother's, husband's, or friend's. Make sure your goal or goals are right for you, and go for it.

Next, understand that you can only achieve a goal if your intention turns into action. Nothing can happen without actual implementation; that is why it is so important to set practical goals. The action will never take place if your goals are too overwhelming. So be practical. Your goal may simply be to become more active by taking relaxed walks with the dog. That's a great starting point and an attainable goal — one that will point you in the right direction. Think long and hard about what direction you want to take to gain health and balanced fitness. Without question, it will involve commitment, time, and persistence. However, once you've zeroed in on your specific goals, it will empower you to begin taking active steps in the right direction.

JOURNAL TO COMMITMENT

By now, you can see the need for realistic, personal goal setting and for taking action to ensure your long-term success. What comes next is commitment. You can set all the goals you want, but if you're not willing to commit yourself to the process, it won't work. But if you are committed to seeing your desires become reality, you will succeed.

My most successful clients are the ones who make every effort to improve the quality of their lives with a step-by-step plan I offer: the S.U.R.E. system. This system helps you to create clear goals and actions, which sets you up for long-term success. By using this system and journaling every step of the way, you will be able to set your path and make adjustments as needed. So take out your journal and write at the top of a new page "My Goals for Success." Beneath that heading, list the system as follows:

> **S**: Is your goal specific?
> **U**: Do you understand the work involved in your goal?
> **R**: Is your goal realistic?
> **E**: Are you enthusiastic about your program?

Now comes a challenging part, applying this system to your goals. It may be tough at first to figure out your true desires, and that's fine. Think about it for a day, even a week, and when you're ready, begin listing your goals. They may consist of reducing the risk of disease or being healthy enough to play ball with your grand-children. You may only have one right now, and that's also fine. List others as you think of them. After a week or two, look at your list and prioritize them. Be realistic. Preventing diabetes needs to be more of a priority than fitting into a pair of pants; if it's not, it should be. Rome wasn't built in a day, so start with your first goal and focus only on that. If you start with too much you'll be overwhelmed and become paralyzed. Now you're ready to apply the S.U.R.E. system to see if your goal is appropriate for you right now. As you go along, feel free to keep adjusting, elaborating, or reevaluating your goal.

The first step is **S**: be *specific*. The more specific you are about your goals, the more you'll be able to weed out anything that isn't about your goal. Then set a date for reaching it, which will help to prevent procrastination and encourage you to look at the practicality of your goal. If you state that you want to lose ten pounds in four months to be healthy and energetic for a trip over-seas, that will be an easier goal to follow than just want-ing to lose weight. You'll be less motivated if your goal is too general.

If your goal seems too general to you, expand it into a subset of goals, or mini-goals. I like using a pyramid to prioritize my goals. First I draw a pyramid, then I divide it into six separate parts and begin listing my general goals at the bottom. Then I move some goals into the next segment and the next until I've come to the top, where I put my most important goal. It's always interesting to see what goal ends up at the top; you may be surprised. Most likely it will be a goal that you feel the most passionate about. And the more passionate you feel about your goal, the more likely you will be to carry it through. Last year, when I went through the S.U.R.E. steps, I would put running a marathon at the top. I had wanted to run a marathon for a long time, and I felt quite passionate about turning this dream into a reality. When I turned it into a true goal, I was ready to take action and commit to seeing it through. It was a bit overwhelming, but I did it, and it turned out to be a wonderful experience.

Now you are ready to move to the next step, **U**: *understand.* Do you understand the time commitment and possible financial, mental, and physical commitment that you'll need to reach this goal? If your specific goal is to improve your health for your trip in June, are you giving yourself adequate time? Or are you putting unnecessary stress on yourself to do something that isn't right for you? If you're planning to walk every day for six weeks have you taken your current health status into consideration? Do you understand the physical demands that the goal you've set requires? If the answer is no, go back to your goal and adjust it so that it works for you. Rather than saying you'll walk every day for six weeks, ask a health professional for advice about what's safe and reasonable for you.

Exercise programs strictly for weight loss often begin with only the end in mind. Investigating the steps necessary to getting there is rarely a consideration but is vital to the success or failure of your goal. It could be compared to getting into your car with the desire to go to Europe. You may not realize it's unreasonable until you reach the coast! So be sure you understand all that is involved in reaching your goals. I've seen too many people let their good intentions fall by the wayside because they didn't realize all that was involved with the goals they chose.

The next step, **R**, is similar: be *realistic*. Setting unrealistic goals is the number-one reason why crash diet and exercise programs fail. One example might be working out to achieve a perfectly flat tummy. If gravity has set in or you've had children, there is little chance you will ever have a perfectly flat stomach. And if you are realistic in your goal-setting step, you will save yourself a lot of aggravation. Why not shoot for stronger legs or lowering your blood pressure? Or eating more fruit and drinking more water? Those sound far more realistic, don't they? And they involve a lot less hassle both mentally and physically.

Now you're at the final step, **E**: *enthusiasm*. As you

look over your goals, are you enthusiastic about the possibilities? Do you look forward to the steps you'll take in order to make them happen? Or do you look at your goals and immediately feel defeated or over-whelmed? If it's the latter, then it's time to go back to step one and reevaluate your goal. Is it specific? Is it realistic? Does it fit in with your lifestyle? Is it what you really want? If you don't necessarily feel defeated but your goal doesn't do much for you, you may have set your goal too low. Goals need to be challenging enough to even warrant being defined as goals. Where's the motivation if there's no challenge? Remember what I mentioned earlier about passion? You've got to be pas-sionate to carry something through. So make sure the goal or goals you've set forth spark excitement and con-fidence.

KEEPING ON TRACK

At this point you've listed your goal or goals. Maybe you've created your own pyramid so you can home in on the goal you feel most passionate about. You've care-fully looked over your goals and have analyzed the kinds of commitment that will be involved in reaching them. If you've done all of the above, now it's time to look over your stated goals with sheer determination and hope.

Look at your journal every day. Make sure your listed

goals or goal keep you excited. If not, go back to the beginning of this chapter and reread it. With this process, whether it involves exercise, nutrition, a job, or a vacation, you're on a continuous journey that offers you the opportunity to learn what is just right for you. If you've gone through your S.U.R.E steps, you know you've set a goal that is appropriate for you. You are ready to flourish rather than be defeated by some unrealistic program with distorted expectations. One of the great things about becoming a goal setter is that your goals continue to change as you progress. If for some reason your stated goal is becoming too difficult to attain, just fall back on your S.U.R.E system. Maybe the time or expense became too much. But instead of walking away feeling like a failure, just readjust your goal until it's right for you. And that is what it's all about: what is right for you. Your goals are uniquely yours; they will direct your life according to your dreams, desires, and passions. Generic programs don't work because you are not generic. You are one of a kind, an exceptional individual who deserves the right to participate fully in the direction you give your life. With appropriate goal setting you will see that the desires of your heart can become the reality of your future.

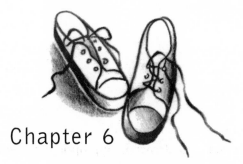

Chapter 6

PUTTING IT ALL TOGETHER

Life is easy if you never take a risk

Throughout this book I have emphasized the importance of avoiding the too-much-too-soon trap of unrealistic dieting and exercise programs. If you try to reconstruct your life overnight, it's going to be so overwhelming that you'll give up and go back to square one. This book (as I hope you know by now) is not about achieving perfection but about working your way toward being the best you. If the goals you've set for yourself are realistic, then you'll succeed in meeting them. And once you've succeeded with one goal, each successive goal will become easier and easier. In this chapter I'll discuss the normal obstacles that occur no matter how dedicated you are to maintaining a balanced lifestyle with a focus on body, mind, and spirit. Unrealistic diets aren't the only reason we feel we fail, and inactive lifestyles aren't the only reason we feel unfulfilled.

As you read this chapter, feel confident in the understanding that you will never achieve perfect balance, but that you can come darned close. And coming close is quite an accomplishment in itself. Speaking for myself, sometimes when I am having a really strong exercise week, my nutrition becomes more of a challenge, or vice versa. I always figure that as long as I keep up something positive for myself, I'm headed in the right direction. As long as my health is in the forefront of all my decisions, I will rarely go off the deep end with no exercise or binges of chocolate or high-sodium foods. I've come to realize, as you will, that it's just not worth feeling that lousy. I know now what puts limits on my effectiveness: it's not exercising and not eating well, and then feeding myself negative mental messages.

Because of my job, some people have said to me, "Oh, I bet you never splurge on ice cream," or whatever food seems most "sinful" to them. They often seem relieved, even surprised, when I tell them I've been known to knock off a hot fudge sundae more than once! It's important to understand that a day of inactivity or some overindulgence with food is not a reason to punish yourself. Keep the circumstances in mind. Were you at a party? Did you have a family crisis? Was it a holiday? Or did you just need to splurge on a special treat? That's where your nutrition log, where you track your emotions and physical responses to your nutrition as well, comes in handy. If you felt guilty about not exercising or not eating right, acknowledge it, understand that tomorrow is another day, and move on. The more you punish yourself for not eating right or exercising enough, the less room you leave for understanding that perfection isn't part of reality. The more you accept reality instead of perfection, the greater the possibilities for getting closer to balance.

DEALING WITH OBSTACLES TO EXERCISE

We all know how things can happen that end up changing all our good intentions. One day we're exercising and eating well, and the next day we can't seem to stop eating. Whether it's a crisis in the family, a seasonal change, or a job transition, suddenly we're off track.

There is little in our society that is conducive to healthy living. With the vast array of fast-food restaurants and our increasingly sedentary lifestyles, keeping on a healthy track can be one of the biggest challenges we face. For this reason, it's more common than not to find oneself sedentary six months after setting up a well-intentioned exercise program. But rather than focusing on all the times we weren't able to stick with it, let's figure out what exactly slips us up and what we can do to break through those obstacles to create a long-term healthy lifestyle.

As I've stressed earlier in this book, if you are currently inactive, you must start the exercise part of your program off slowly. Starting off too hot and heavy has proved to be the demise of many a good intention. Whether you want to start with a walk around the block, a stroll to the end of the driveway, or a mile-long hike, it makes no difference. What matters is that it's a comfortable starting point for you.

I'm a firm believer that those of us living in the Midwest and the northern parts of the country have a far greater challenge when it comes to maintaining consistent exercise programs. If you're a seasoned athlete, changes in the weather pose little if any challenge. For the rest of us, weather changes can throw us completely off track. Parents know how important it is to keep a child's life structured, to provide a feeling of security. When that structure suddenly changes it can be very disturbing. The same goes for the novice exerciser who has been walking for three months when suddenly subzero temperatures hit. Unless she was given some direction on how to prepare herself, the freezing temperature can completely derail her.

Not only can changes in weather pose a challenge, but changes in lifestyle can throw us off course as well. When our lifestyle is altered, everything needs to shift to accommodate the change. So the best tip I can give you is to have a plan. If you begin your first walking program in July, and you know that come September the kids will be in school, why not begin August by plotting out your new schedule and listing activities to accommodate it. If you know it's going to be too cold to walk outside, consider taking an exercise class. Visit some classes, maybe with a friend, to get an idea of what they're like before signing up — remember my experience? If the class idea is a turnoff, then I would encourage purchasing a treadmill. In fact, anyone who experiences extreme winter weather should own a treadmill; it can get you through the winter until the weather is temperate again. If you have no interest in owning a treadmill or it's not in the budget now, a videotape may be your best bet. (See chapter 7 for some recommendations.)

Come January, you'll again be thrown into a lifestyle change. The kids will be home on vacation, your work may slow down a bit, the gyms will be packed, and so forth. I would encourage you to start making contingency plans by December 1. Then when April rolls around, begin preparing yourself for the new summer schedules and activities. If you can get through an entire year of adjusting your exercise program, you will become a successful, long-term exerciser. You know all too well that seasons greatly affect your exercise programs. By being better prepared, you have a better chance of making the transition more easily. I'm not saying that simply by planning ahead you'll fall right into the next season without a hitch — on the contrary. But through trial and error you'll soon find what works and allows you to stay in touch with your newfound program.

PERSONAL CRISIS, NUTRITION, AND EXERCISE

If I had a dollar for every time a client strayed from her program due to a family crisis or a life transition, I'd be a wealthy woman. Without a doubt major crises such as divorce, death, becoming an empty-nester, and so forth will take us to uncharted emotional territory. And when we find ourselves without a map, we generally fall back on something that feels familiar and comfortable, such as eating "comfort food" or sitting on the couch and channel surfing.

When a crisis hits, we never know just how we'll react. Sometimes instead of eating too much we starve ourselves, because the knot in our stomach keeps us from feeling hungry. Often we neglect what seems least important to us at the time, which generally means exercise or good nutrition. But I tell my clients that during a crisis it's more important than ever to continue your exercise and nutrition programs, because they will both enable you to handle the crisis better, especially when combined. Exercise will help you work off excess stress and give you more energy with which to deal with problems, while good nutrition keeps you strong and helps prevent mood swings.

A woman whose husband has left her will obviously be thrown into crisis. She may react by overeating or she may stop exercising as a way of punishing herself for not being good enough. Or at the other end of the spectrum, she may starve herself in an attempt to become desirable again. In a situation like that many women feel powerless. But the best way to reclaim power is by strengthening your body and mind through exercise and eating right. Often the grief is so overwhelming that nothing else seems to matter, including taking care of ourselves. Acknowledge that grief with the help of a counselor, and try to value yourself enough to maintain your physical health. During a crisis, it may help to reread chapter 5 for some encouragement to keep on your journey toward healthy living.

HOLIDAYS, SPECIAL EVENTS, AND NUTRITION

Be honest: How many times have you vowed not to eat dessert or not to overeat at a party or wedding you're attending? And on the other side of the coin, how many holiday meals have you finished while mentally reprimanding yourself for overeating? Neither of these approaches work very well. Vowing not to eat treats at a special event leaves us open to feeling guilty if we do choose to indulge in that special desert, or to feel deprived if we resist all treats. Ultimately, enjoying yourself at a special event means going prepared.

I always advise my clients to eat something before going to a party. How many times have you starved yourself all day long because you knew you were going to a party at night? And what happens? You end up scarfing enough food to feed a small country because you went to the party ravenous. As stated above, it's not a crime to treat yourself to a special "goodie." It's when you vow not to eat anything and you end up eating everything that you're left feeling mentally and physically miserable. When I attend a wedding or a holiday party, I always allow myself one dessert, and I make sure to pick my favorite. At a wedding buffet, one spoonful of everything (I mean a soup spoon not a serving spoon!) is a way to sample different yummy foods without overeating. Sometimes I share my plate with my husband or a friend. If you're still hungry, opt for the veggies and fruit. But of course, if you do overindulge, it's not the end of the world, and it doesn't mean the end of all your hard work, either. Obsessing about overeating can lead you to eat more just to punish yourself. But there's no need for that; tomorrow is another day.

TRAVELING FIT

Keeping your exercise and nutrition in balance while on a vacation or business trip can also be a challenge. If you're staying in a hotel, keep in mind that many hotels offer exercise facilities. Not everyone is comfortable using them, however, and if that's the case with you, then try a workout in your room. Here's a sample hotel room program. Keep in mind that if you're just starting out, do fewer repetitions: Begin with jogging or marching in place for three minutes, do thirty sit-ups, then march or jog for three more minutes, do as many push-ups as you can do (if you're a beginner, do push-ups against the wall), march or jog in place for three minutes again, and then do twelve forward lunges for each leg. (To perform a lunge, stand with feet a shoulder width apart, take a big step forward with one foot while keeping the other foot in place and slowly bend both knees until the front thigh is parallel to the floor. Push back to the starting position with the front foot and alternate the lead foot. If you feel pain anywhere, stop! Keep your back straight and make sure your front knee does not go past your toes. If you're a beginner, do very shallow lunges to avoid knee injury. As you get stronger you can lunge deeper.) Finish the workout with three more minutes of marching or jogging in place. If you go through this program once, you've spent about twelve to fifteen minutes exercising, and if you go through it twice, you've completed thirty minutes. There are many other options, but I find this is a great place to start.

As for your eating, while you're on the road you'll have to decide where and when you want to make the call to monitor your nutrition. For my clients who take their kids to the Disney parks, eating well is always a challenge. Though there are places to get salads, many of them usually grab whatever the kids are eating and call it a meal. I would encourage you to keep fruit in a backpack or travel case, or you can order a grilled chicken sandwich with a side salad. If you snack on nutritious foods, you will have less desire to pig out on junk food. And since we're forced to eat out while traveling (unless we're staying with relatives) it's good to keep some eating-out tips in mind: When you order a salad, always ask for the dressing on the side or you'll find your salad swimming in fatty dressing. Always avoid sautéed foods, since anything sautéed will be very high in fat and calories, and opt for something grilled or broiled instead. Try to limit your intake of alcohol, because alcoholic drinks are calorie heavy and nutrient light. Furthermore, you tend to eat more when you drink.

And the last tip: don't eat too much bread! When it comes to eating at restaurants, I must admit that my biggest pitfall is that bread basket! I can quite easily knock off one of those mini loaves of bread in one sitting. And if the bread is warm, forget about it, it's mine, all mine! But the truth is that eating bread will add an incredible amount of extra calories to my meal without my even being aware. While in deep conversation, I keep nibbling on the bread, and before I know it, it's gone. The end result is that I'm unable to enjoy my meal, which would have been much more nutritious for me, because I've filled up on bread. So take it from one who knows: Limit yourself to one piece before your meal and one with, or eliminate it all together.

OVERCOMING MENTAL OBSTACLES

Now that I've covered some common challenges to maintaining good eating and exercise habits, I'd like to move on to discussing some challenges to maintaining good mental habits as well. For starters, dieting and exercise failures trigger depression and destructive mental messages. A good way to prevent that dynamic is to keep your motivation level high and to follow your goal-setting strategy. We need to keep focused on long-term positive transformation. Think about a great athlete and the years of training it took to get where she is. Ponder planting a tree and the time and nurturing it takes until it finally bears fruit. Or the evolution of a great musician and the painstaking hours spent polishing symphonies so that we can enjoy beautiful music.

Time heals all wounds and allows the creation of

positive growth. All this means that we must create a personal image that we can be comfortable with through patience, persistence, and perspective. During your transition into healthy living, you will begin to understand the time and work it will take to reach your goals. And invariably, fit or unfit, you will encounter obstacles along the way. There isn't a week that passes that I'm not thrown a curve ball and need to adjust my schedule or my exercise routine. It's feeding yourself positive messages that can push you through to the other side.

One of the many obstacles we encounter on the path to healthy living is the comparison game. But playing this game seriously gets in the way of creating positive mental messages for ourselves. During high school, when I was battling with weight issues, I constantly looked at everyone else wishing desperately to have their bodies. But there was no way I could ever look like them. The road to self-acceptance can be a long one, but it's certainly worthwhile. It took me a long time to understand that my body's design was predetermined by my genes. When I finally began to grasp this concept, I was able to work on the things that were within reason for me. Losing weight to feel better, not to look "perfect" became manageable. Instead of wanting to change things that were simply out of my grasp, I was better able to understand and respect my limitations and focus on all I could achieve.

Imagine for a moment if every woman in the world who is currently dieting stopped simultaneously! It would drastically change the attitude of the women in this world. They could only think positive thoughts and involve themselves in positive projects. They would stop thinking about weight or diet. I challenge you to cast aside those confining thoughts about weight loss and perfection and instead to focus on making positive changes. I challenge you to give up the notion of ever having a completely flat belly. I challenge you to give up the notion that if you're not a size six, you'll be a national embarrassment. Finally, I challenge you to believe that you can be and do anything you choose as long as you place your health at the forefront of all your decisions.

ACKNOWLEDGE ALL THAT YOU HAVE

Each time I work with a client, I ask them what their body was able to do that week that amazed them? Or I'll ask them, what part of your body are you most aware of and appreciate and why? By focusing on these positive images, you begin to understand the amazing abilities you possess. I try not to let a day pass without appreciating some aspect of my body. I prize my ability to hear, speak, or see. I never take for granted that I am able to take my stairs two at a time. I notice individuals with physical limitations and think about their challenges. A gentleman at my church is in a wheelchair.

Each Sunday I watch him wheel down to communion and then back up a very steep incline to return to his spot by the pew. One day I was sitting in church "PMSing" and looking down at my protruding belly thinking, "Oh, you fatty." But when my eyes connected with his, I underwent a serious attitude adjustment. Here I was obsessing about a little fat, while this gentlemen is challenged every day by tasks as simple as getting dressed. The point I'm trying to make is that we may not be perfect, but if we take time to appreciate our gifts and abilities, we will fill our minds with positive and appreciative thoughts.

Do you believe that you can choose how you will meet each day? Beginning your day with positive messages can get your day off to a fantastic start. You can begin by telling yourself each morning before you get out of bed, "Today I will treat my body to nutritious food, I will provide my body with positive movement, and I will remind myself of all the blessings that are uniquely mine." By starting each day this way you are validating your worthiness and acknowledging how blessed your life is.

The more you strive to improve upon the talents that are uniquely yours, the better off you will be. Focus on improving the things that continue to make you the very best you. Wanting to be a certain size or shape (unless it's for health reasons) will not change the core of who you are. After I had lost all the weight I had wanted to lose, I was certain that along with those forty plus pounds would go all my bad habits and all my challenges in life and my new exterior would ensure a new me. But reality set in as I realized the weight was gone, but that I was still there.

Losing weight and exercising improved my heart and lungs and gave me more strength and day-to-day energy, but it didn't change the core of who I was. I had to appreciate not only my physical self but all that I was doing to improve the quality of my life. Recognizing the changes I was making kept my desire for healthy living a reality. The changes you are beginning to make are fantastic. Recognize your willingness to change the habits that limit your abilities and see your life slowly come together. Isn't it great what you are able to do?

HEALTHY RELATIONSHIPS RESULT IN HEALTHY LIVING

Though many of the changes you'll be making will be made by you, having a support system can dramatically affect your inspiration to continue on your positive path. Part of making positive choices about your health includes those whom you choose to involve in your life. Mutually rewarding relationships are a necessary component of positive living. I'm sure I'm not the only one who has been involved in relationships that were damaging both emotionally and mentally. Unhealthy relationships are just as bad for you as sitting down with a pie and knocking off the whole thing. I'm not just talking about romantic relationships, I'm talking about friends and other family members also. Negative vibes create a negative environment, something we can all do without. Make it a goal to seek out those people who move you forward on your path to better living, not set you back.

As a child, I had a very negative home environment, but we had family friends with whom I could stay with on the weekends. These people had an incredible impact on my life. They encouraged me to see the good person that I was, and they believed in me. All children need that kind of support and unconditional love. As I moved forward in my life and away from those friends, I dabbled in unstable relationships but always returned to mutually respecting relationships. Strong, healthy relationships of any kind encourage healthy choices. Think about the times when you were involved in bad relationships; what kind of mental or physical abuse did you sustain? Now think about the impact of positive relationships on your life and how confident they have made you feel.

I have the unbelievable good fortune to have married a saint! I first have to credit myself with making a good choice (we're allowed to credit ourselves with good choices once in a while!). Second, I credit my happy marriage to the fact that I want good things for myself and for my health. And relationships are a huge part of our overall health, because they involve so much of our energy, both physically and mentally. A negative relationship creates a negative lifestyle, and a positive relationship creates a positive lifestyle. It's that simple. And you are the only one who can make that choice.

Unhealthy relationships can be obstacles on our journey toward healthy living. But with all that you've learned thus far with goal setting — choosing realistic exercise and nutrition choices — you can approach those obstacles better prepared. My marriage is fantastic, but my husband and I have had our challenges, without a doubt. But it's much easier to handle those challenges with someone you respect than with someone who belittles the decisions you make to improve yourself. By surrounding yourself with those that believe in you, trust you, and love you, you'll have an unbelievable support system that will enable you to stay on your path toward balanced, happy living.

JOURNAL TO FULFILLMENT

As you learn to appreciate yourself during this transition to healthy living, it may help to put in writing the things that are uniquely, wonderfully you. Writing them down somehow makes them count. Rather than just being a thought, it becomes authentic. I'd like you to take out your journal again. I want you to open it to the very last page and turn your journal upside down. This is where you'll start. You've been keeping track of all the changes you're making to your lifestyle, and now it's time to keep track of what you like about yourself. To move forward with healthy living, first you must uncover all your great qualities.

At the top of the page, write the heading "Five Physical Traits I Have That Are Special." Then list at least five things — though there are many more you've yet to discover! Maybe you especially like your eyes. Maybe you're proud of your strong arms. Your next heading will be "Five Mental Traits I Have That Are Special." Again, list at least five traits. Maybe you're a good writer or a voracious reader or a wonderful teacher. Next write the heading "Five Things That I Treasure," and again, list at least five items. Maybe you'd like to include a person you're close to, or a special gift you received from someone. Think of anything that is special to you. Finally, I want you to list "Five Things That I Will Do to Improve the Quality of My Life." Examples might be sleep fifteen minutes more each night, eat at least one piece of fruit every day, donate two hours a week to volunteer work, walk every day, and so on. You may not be able to come up with five items right away for every category, and that's okay. Fill them in as you are able and if you go past five, that's great too!

MOVING BEYOND LIMITATIONS

As you begin to uncover things about yourself that you had forgotten or never recognized, suddenly the numbers on the bathroom scale will seem pretty insignificant. If enough women were able to cast aside their obsession with those numbers and to instead seek out their true talents, they would be much more likely to attain their personal best. The result? I believe that we would experience a major growth in contributions by women to our society and that there would be many more female leaders and role models.

I am firmly convinced that women stay in the shadows because they are stifled by feelings of inadequacy. We need to start living our lives according to what we find acceptable about ourselves and not according to someone else's ideas about what's acceptable. To that end, I would like you to use the following line as a positive statement to make to yourself each day. Write it on a piece of paper and put it on your fridge, in your billfold, or in your purse. But read it every day:

It's not a matter of fat or thin, it's how my heart beats, my mind thinks, and my body moves.

I would not be giving you the whole story if all I talked about was exercise and eating healthful foods. Your health is about so much more than that, it's about the essence of you and what makes you the best you can be. This book is about finding a well-rounded fitness program, one that encompasses physical, mental, and spiritual health, to help you feel that you're the best you can be. Your life comes along but once, and it is yours to embrace, explore, and evolve in. You are here for a reason, and although you may not know what that reason is, as long as you expect the best of yourself by doing things that resonate with you, you will be the best you that you can be. As long as your goals are yours alone and realistic for you, you will reach and exceed them every time.

As a child I was told that girls don't need to go to college because there's nothing they need to learn except how to fold laundry and make dinner. Yes, ladies, just writing that makes the hair on the back of my neck stand up. But I bring it up because if that was all I ever expected of myself, I would never be where I am now. I have always been a dreamer (even during those tough times), an optimist, and a hopeless romantic. Against all odds, I have held onto those traits. Along the way I learned that unrealistic dieting and exercise programs are simply limitations to the opportunity to grow, discover, and teach others. The more I move beyond the limitations I and others have set for me, the more every day surprises me with yet another opportunity to learn and grow. You are an incredible gift, put on this planet to make a difference. I am certain that the limitations you cast aside now will allow you to unfold and contribute to the quality of your own life as well as to the quality of others.

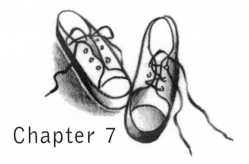

Chapter 7

A FITNESS RESOURCE GUIDE

Any gadget promising fast and easy weight loss will be obsolete next year!

One of the most confusing aspects of exploring diet, health, and fitness options is the incessant contradictory information with which we're all bombarded. One magazine ad says "lose fifteen pounds in fifteen days," while another warns that "a fifteen-pound weight loss in less than two weeks may be hazardous to your health!" Or how about fitness equipment: one TV commercial offers the best results, while another suggests that their machine is the only one on the market guaranteed to give you results. It can be incredibly difficult to choose what's right for you as well as what is safe and effective.

Most companies sell their products by telling us what we want to hear. The supposedly unrivaled piece of equipment will provide you with that flat tummy you've been seeking. The commercials and ads for diet programs shout out, "You can have the body you've always wanted!" Naturally we buy things that promise to make losing weight and exercising easier. We're all looking for an easy answer to our fitness dilemmas. But there is no easy answer. Furthermore, the fitness arena is constantly changing, so even if you've been through years of schooling and have a degree in physiology, it's hard to keep up. The same goes for nutrition. One month we read that margarine is better than butter, then we are told that although butter has more fat, it's safer to use than margarine.

We're all trying to locate the ideal — the ideal piece of equipment, the ideal nutrition program, the ideal running shoe. But what we must keep in mind is that one person's ideal is another person's disaster. Thus, it's important that you find what is right for you and you only. It's always important to take general information you get from the TV or from a magazine ad with a grain of salt until you get more information. In this chapter I will be providing you with some very specific fitness resources. But before I do, let me first give you a list of things to keep in mind whenever you read an article, see a commercial, or contemplate buying a piece of exercise equipment. These tips will help you make sensible choices about your health program.

When a new diet is introduced, the first and only question you need to ask yourself is, "Is this something I can live with for the rest of my life?" If the answer is no, then the diet is inappropriate and will probably leave you seeking yet another unrealistic program and feeling like a failure. This is where so many of us miss the boat on learning how to eat right. We start a diet with strict guidelines, never considering the long-term consequences. Women in this country average three to four diets a year, because they don't consider whether they can stay on their diets for a month, let alone a lifetime. It's so much better to gradually change habits so that in a year you'll be in a much better place than you would've been had you started that unrealistic program.

If the nutritional intake for a diet is less than 1,500 calories a day, you will gain all the weight back once you get off the program. This probably isn't news for those of you who have experienced the yo-yo syndrome. Eating less than 1,500 calories a day is not only dangerous, it is also totally unrealistic for a well-balanced diet and a practical lifestyle. Sure, you'll drop weight if you're eating 1,200 calories a day, but once you leave the restricted program, the weight comes back. Again, diets promising you a dramatic initial weight loss are teaching you nothing about long-term healthy eating. All you're learning is that if you deprive yourself you'll lose weight, and it's not that likely you'll survive deprivation for very long.

Whether it's about exercise, diet, or equipment, if anything makes a promise or guarantee, it's probably not worth picking up. This is true especially if it guarantees results in a ridiculous amount of time, such as losing fifteen pounds in fifteen days. And how many times have we seen those late-night shopping networks selling pieces of equipment and touting fantastic results? Do you notice how they always have some buff babe demonstrating and making it look so easy? For most of us, starting anything new is never easy, so don't be sucked in by beautiful women telling you what you can do to look just like them. If you think you can, refer back to the introduction of this book.

Does the product or program address your health? I have yet to see any ads for diet pills, diet programs, or miracle exercise machines mention anything about health. If you're researching a diet program, ask yourself, does the program follow realistic, safe guidelines? Does it encourage exercise along with the program? Is there any evidence that suggests that your health comes first?

If you're considering buying a piece of equipment, ask yourself the following: Is it something you like to do? Is it complicated or fairly self-explanatory? Can you do it on your own or might you need some help? I can't tell you how many seminars I've done in which I ask for a show of hands for all those who own an exercise bike. Seventy-five percent of the audience raises their hands. Then I ask them how many of them actually like to ride bikes, and maybe two people raise their hands. Well if you didn't like bike riding before you bought the bike, you won't like it after. If you've never rowed a boat, why buy a rowing machine? Or if you purchase a piece of equipment that would challenge an engineer, you'll never follow through with using it. I can't tell you how many homes I've gone to and seen gorgeous equipment that has gone unused. Why? Because it's too complicated and because the owners don't know where to start. So look for equipment that you'll enjoy, something that appeals to your abilities and fitness level. For example, if you've never done any exercise, a treadmill is a great choice because everyone knows how to walk. Whatever you choose, explore it further by getting all the information you can. You can always refer to *Consumer Reports* magazine for quality issues or consult fitness experts about safety and effectiveness.

The only true way to improve health and become fit is through a careful process that involves time, patience, and education. Ingrain that sentence in your mind. It will prevent you from jumping on anything that looks too good to be true. Nothing of quality can be attained overnight, and the same goes for your health. If it's fast and easy, then it's not quality information or results you're getting.

The vast array of magazines, videotapes, books, equipment, exercise clothing and so on can be very confusing. In an effort to guide you toward quality information and products, I have compiled my selections of items you may need to get you on, and keep you on, the road to health and fitness. This is not a complete list: If I haven't mentioned a particular item or magazine, that doesn't mean I'm denouncing it, it simply means it's not appropriate for this list or that I don't know about it. The following list reflects suggestions I pass on to my clientele. They find that these suggestions help them to make better decisions about their exercise program, keep up with fitness trends, and increase their motivation during times of struggle.

MAGAZINES

Before investing in a subscription, first decide what you're looking for in a magazine. You can go to your local library and leaf through some or buy a few from a local store. Do you want information strictly about fitness, or would you like some nutrition tips and recipes as well? Are you seeking serious, medical research and study results or real-life success stories?

The magazines I've listed here are the ones that I feel are the best choices if you want up-to-date information about health and fitness issues. And rather than insinuating that being healthy means being thin, most of the magazines I've selected portray health in all sizes, shapes, lifestyles, and attitudes — reality!

Prevention (Rodale Press). When I think of health and fitness magazines, *Prevention* tops the list with its ability to provide information for everyone from the most sedentary person to the physically challenged to the master athlete. The magazine is the same size as *Reader's Digest,* so it's easy to handle and carry. The articles are always concise, skillfully written, and well researched, and the writers for the most part specialize in the field they are writing about. Because health and fitness information always changes, *Prevention* does a great job of updating information and provides data from different perspectives. It covers a wide array of information without being overwhelming. I'm always able to read this magazine cover to cover in a reasonable amount of time. This is a smart magazine for smart people who deserve good information about current health and fitness issues.

Walking (RD Walking). The comment I hear most frequently from my clients is, "I hate to run. Please don't tell me I have to run to lose weight!" I always assure my clients that running is a personal choice, not my choice.

It goes back to what I said in chapter 3: you've got to find the exercise that motivates you to continue. Maybe walking is more your cup of tea; both walking and running are calorie-burning activities. *Walking* magazine is appropriate for various levels of walkers, and there's even some good stuff for us die-hard runners. It addresses issues of concern among women regarding the newest health and fitness crazes. *Walking* often features articles about special getaways that offer plenty for walkers. I especially love the "walking shorts" section at the beginning, which provides bits and pieces of health and fitness information, ranging from the newest breakthrough in breast cancer research to the latest exercise trend. *Walking* covers mind, body, and spirit and is also a great forum for highlighting practical fitness regimes. The wonderful stories about walkers are almost enough to get me to trade in my running shoes for a great walk through a Midwest forest preserve. The beauty of it is, I don't have to trade in my running shoes, I just alternate my running with the serenity of an invigorating walk. I recommend *Walking* magazine to those of you who like to walk and have been turned off by the "beautiful people" magazines. It leaves out the fluff and is adept at motivating even the most inexperienced walker. *Walking* gives you ideas about how to gauge your walking program, how to invigorate it a bit, how to provide variety, and so much more.

Fitness (G & J, U.S.A. Publishing). When it comes to the plethora of beauty magazines, I find that *Fitness* magazine does the best job at combining beauty with reality. The magazine features a variety of models of different body types and looks and is careful not to shove the "thin is best" message down your throat. I love the many snippets of fitness, health, and nutrition information at the beginning of every issue, especially if I'm crunched for time. Granted, some of the articles are fluffy, but for the most part the magazine does a nice job of combining the polish of *Shape* and *Cosmopolitan* with well-written articles and photos that provide accurate exercise options. I have particularly enjoyed when the editors have shared their personal fitness successes and struggles. In addition, it's a nice magazine for those who are already active and seeking updates to their fitness programs. There are great articles on nutrition that explore the trends and provide a thumbs-up or thumbs-down analysis. Other stories may focus on depression, spirituality, divorce, and so on. Fitness is a well-rounded magazine for all fitness levels.

Cooking Light (Southern Living). *Cooking Light* has been a part of my life for ten years, almost since its first issue. It's been great watching how it has grown and evolved. When I started receiving this magazine, 90 percent of it was on cooking and 10 percent was on fitness and nutrition tips. Now it is beautifully put together with fitness and medical information in the first half and the seemingly unending, delicious, heart-healthy recipes in the second half of the magazine. One of the reasons I was initially drawn to this magazine was the fact that I wanted to begin to cook differently for my family, and it was difficult to find decent, practical, yummy recipes. *Cooking Light* offered tried-and-true family favorites and turned them into healthier family favorites. My cooking has evolved right along with this magazine. Rarely do I find recipes that are less than delicious, and most are easy to prepare. Each year they put out a color cookbook including the best of their recipes. But personally, I like clipping the recipes and laminating them for my personal *Cooking Light* recipe box! You can't go wrong with this magazine and now you can access the magazine online at www.cookinglight.com.

BOOKS

New books about health and fitness are published every day. When purchasing a fitness or nutrition book, I like to stick to basics. I don't care for any book that provides a twelve-week or twelve-step solution to years of exercise and nutrition "mismanagement." I like information that is timeless as opposed to trendy, that is realistic and appropriate for most people. Some movie stars have come out with their own beauty and health books, and while it's interesting to read their stories, the truth of the matter is their lives and our lives are very different. Try to look for books that seem to be written for the masses and generally include information that is safe, up to date, and user friendly. As with the magazines, if there are promises of perfect bodies, seek elsewhere. This doesn't mean that exploring a new avenue isn't a good idea. If something piques your interest, pick it up; it may be great for you. But my advice in general is to read things that are applicable to your lifestyle and personality. So, here are a few of my recommendations:

Strong Women Stay Young by Miriam Nelson, Ph.D. (Bantam Books, 1998). Finally, a book that addresses head-on the need for practical weight training for women. There are a number of weight-training books out there, but few of them are geared toward those who really need to be educated about the importance of weight training. They tend to be body-builder books, ten-weeks-to-a-better-body books, which are fine if you're already weight training or active. But if you're just learning, this book provides timeless information. It's not a gimmicky or quick-and-easy guide to eternal youth. Rather, it focuses on the importance of weight training for women and explains it in terms that make sense for every fitness level. The drawings portray real bodies rather than the airbrushed "beauties" of other exercise books. *Strong Women Stay Young* addresses common questions about weight training and shares information that is necessary for women to read and retain. I recommend this book to every female client who comes through my door.

Too Busy to Exercise by Porter Shimer (Storey Communications, 1996). This book is useful for both the busy executive who lives in hotel rooms during the week and the house executive who barely has a moment to herself. The author gives great suggestions for time management and exercise. I usually suggest this book to those who are in a pretty regular routine and need some tips on adding more quality and variety to their busy programs. The tips in this book address after-five exercise, at-home exercise, on-the-road exercise, and more. *Too Busy to Exercise* leaves no room for excuses but plenty of room for improving the quality of your time-crunched exercise program.

Nutrition for Women by Elizabeth Sommer, M.A., R.D. (Henry Holt, 1995). This is far and away the best resource for proper nutrition for women. It offers no crazy programs, just accurate, safe information. *Nutrition for Women* covers everything from proper vitamin supplements to healthy brown-bag lunches to eating disorders. The focus in this book is health — yay! It offers a "no frill," honest approach to lifelong healthy eating habits. I also believe that much of the information in this book will be applicable for many years. If you want to be educated on proper nutrition that will keep you on the track to healthy eating, this is the book for you.

Busy Mom's Low Fat Cookbook by Elise M. Griffith (Prima Publishing, 1997). What a find this book was! You may have a hundred healthy cookbooks, but few will include kid-friendly meals like this one. Most of the recipes require minimal prep time and are as pleasing to the eye as they are to the palate. From breakfast goodies to creative lunch suggestions, this is a must for any mother out there who is currently cooking a different meal for each child!

EQUIPMENT

The same rule applies to equipment as to magazines and books. If the company selling the exercise machine makes unrealistic promises, I wouldn't explore it any further. Unlike a book, equipment can be very dangerous if it's inappropriate for you, so be very careful with your selections. And I go crazy when I watch these infomercials pushing a piece of equipment that even Einstein couldn't figure out. Thousands of these so-called "fat-burning" machines are sold every minute. Remember, if it looks complicated on TV, it probably is. Or if some gorgeous babe promises that you too can look just like her after just a couple of weeks on the "ab-b-gone," forget about it. That said, let me share my suggestions for good equipment:

Treadmills. My dream is that one day, every family that owns a computer will also own a treadmill. Treadmills simply provide the movement of walking on a revolving surface. Except, with this piece of equipment, you can speed up, slow down, or increase the incline. With handles to grip for beginners, treadmills are safe and easy to use. Hands down, the treadmill is the piece of equipment most frequently suggested by my staff and me. Whether you're ten or a hundred, the most deconditioned person alive or an elite athlete, you can use it. A treadmill can provide a minimal exercise experience or a kick-your-butt workout. The most commonly asked question is, "How much should I spend?" It depends. If you can afford to spend $1,000 to $2,000 or more on a treadmill, that will buy a beautiful one and it will be money well spent. But I certainly don't want to leave out those who can't afford that much. It's also true that $500 to $800 can get you a decent treadmill that will probably last you five to seven years, maybe longer. At that point you may want to invest more money in your next one. Obviously, spending more money will get you more bells and whistles, a better guarantee, and generally better information from your salesperson. Shop around and try an expensive one, then try a less expensive one and establish what matters most to you. Read *Consumer Reports;* they usually have pretty good information about fitness equipment in their January or

February issues. The best thing about treadmills is that when used properly, they are both safe and easy.

Free Weights. I love free weights (dumb bells) almost as much as I love the treadmill. Why? Because they're a way to bring a health club into your home without spending a fortune. Free weights are a great way to weight train, especially for us smaller women. Often machines don't align with our bodies properly and the risk of injury is increased, but free weights have no height or size limitations. I recommend free weights over a multi-station unit, which allows several exercises on one piece of equipment, for three reasons: cost, space, and ease of use. Form is much easier to establish with free weights than with a multi-station unit. If this all sounds like Greek to you, I suggest reading *Strong Women Stay Young* (see page 131). Given proper training, free weights can be very beneficial. They're an excellent way to develop and improve your muscle strength, prevent or minimize osteoporosis, and so on. You can find free weights just about anywhere, but remember, never start a weight-training program without proper instruction. A videotape doesn't count. The videotape instructor can't see if you've got your wrist bent or your arms too high. It doesn't cost very much to set up an appointment with a certified personal trainer. Not only will they guide you in proper technique with the free weights, they'll also tell you how much weight you should be using as well as what you need to begin a program.

SHOES AND CLOTHING

If you live in the Midwest, your clothing and shoe needs will differ greatly from those of someone living in southern California. I generally encourage quality clothing for healthy, comfortable exercise. Nothing is worse than a cheap exercise bra that rubs your underarms raw or socks that allow your foot to stay moist, resulting in blisters. You can get quality clothing from a number of places, but educate yourself first on what you need. Then decide how much you want to spend. If you are on a limited budget, keep away from exclusive designs and head to your nearest sports equipment chain, where you can find more reasonably priced items.

For starters, every woman should have a quality sports bra. You can find one at a lingerie boutique or a sports store. If you opt for the lingerie boutique, it may cost you more, but you'll be fitted properly. A proper fit can make a huge difference, especially if you're big busted. When it comes to shoes, the only place I can wholeheartedly recommend is Road Runner Sports, which sells both walking and running shoes. The prices seem to be competitive. And their customer service is fantastic! The sales reps will ask you questions about your fitness level and assist you in choosing the best shoe for your needs. Their staff is well educated about their products and can answer just about any question you might have. They'll even answer your questions about proper clothing for your particular climate. Although you can find a variety of shoes at any sports store, please keep in mind that the quality of your shoe is very important. A poor shoe can cause an injury, possibly preventing you from continuing your activities. Quality and proper fit are your top priorities when exploring your shoe options. Road Runner can be found on the web at www.roadrunnersports.com.

When it comes to women's sportswear, Title Nine is a great catalog specializing in women's active wear. Again, they can answer your clothing questions about fabrics and what works best for your region. They offer a great variety of clothing for all body and activity types. They also carry running bras. It's a bit pricey, but again, whatever you buy will carry you through many years. And that's the hope — that you'll need it for many years! Title Nine can also be reached on the web at www.title9sports.com. They have a great selection, and the customer service is above average. Road Runner also carries exercise clothing, and although it's geared more toward the runner, you can find some great gear for winter walking. If price is an issue, again, explore your local sporting goods store and know what attire will work best for your exercise program. I don't want to be too specific because everyone is comfortable in something different. Explore your options, and you'll find what is useful with your program.

VIDEOTAPES

I won't recommend specific videotapes, but I will give you information on what to look out for when selecting one. First of all, check the length. If you're a beginner, you don't want a tape that's ninety minutes long. Then check for level of difficulty; if it's intermediate or advanced and you're a beginner or unable to do anything high impact, keep away from it. My biggest fear when it comes to beginners buying videos is that many people are uneducated about form. I have seen far too many videos that assume the viewer knows what to do. Unfortunately, the result is horrific soreness, injury, or frustration. As I suggested with free weights, hire someone to help you. She or he can help you to identify your limitations and teach you how to modify your movements. I met a woman once who had followed a videotape for three months that had given her chronic arm and knee pain and little in the way of results. The tape was okay, but she had no idea that her form was all wrong, which was causing the injury. Further, the amount of jumping around she did was not appropriate for her fitness level, and she was so out of breath she had to keep stopping, which prevented her from increasing her endurance and strength. There are so many opportunities to injure yourself if you don't know what you're doing. Please don't let that happen. There's a fairly good catalog out called CollageVideo, which lists hundreds of videos reviewed by all levels of fitness enthusiasts. They are rated by level of difficulty and by time. It's a nice way to narrow down what may or may not be appropriate for you. You can view their various selections on the internet at www.collagevideo.com.

WORKOUT MUSIC

I'm sure you're thinking, can't I just turn on the radio or play a favorite CD? Sure, both of those ideas are great, but I have a suggestion that could really make a difference in your workouts. A catalog entitled Workout Music actually develops tapes that are speed appropriate, meaning that if you are currently walking at, say, 3.2 miles an hour on your treadmill, you can buy a tape that has a 3.2 back beat that keeps you at that pace when you're walking outside with your Walkman. That way you don't need to worry about losing the speed that you gained over the winter. If you're a runner, you can buy a tape that keeps you at your running speed. And these tapes come in a great variety of music, from jazz to Motown to top forty. These tapes are great for everyone, from beginners up to the most advanced. Workout Music has expanded to offer music for bikers, walkers, runners, steppers, rollerbladers, and other sports. You can order a catalog by calling 1-800-878-4764 or reach them on the internet at www.clearzone.com.

There are so many choices you can make when it comes to health, fitness, and nutrition accessories, and I hope I've taken some of the confusion out of the process. If you know of any great publications that would be appropriate for a novice, please let me know so that I can add it to my collection of resources. The health and fitness undertaking offers a number of challenges no matter what step of the fitness ladder you're on. Seeking out new ideas and suggestions can help to keep your program fresh and challenging. That's the key to long-term success. I hope that the resources I have provided will enable you to continue safely toward your stated goals. Here's to realistic, healthy living, today and always!

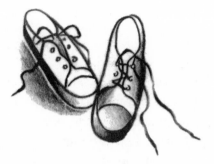

ABOUT THE AUTHOR

A working mother of four children, Nicki Anderson is president and owner of Reality Fitness, Inc., a full-service personal training studio in Naperville, Illinois. She is a certified personal trainer and fitness practitioner and has appeared frequently as a motivational speaker on fitness and on Chicago-area radio and television. Her articles on fitness have appeared in newspapers and national fitness magazines.